Considering Weight-Loss Surgery

A Patient's Guide to Surgery

Second Edition

Considering Weight-Loss Surgery

A Patient's Guide to Surgery

Second Edition

By
Glenn M. Ihde, MD

Order this book online at www.trafford.com
or email orders@trafford.com

Most Trafford titles are also available at major online book retailers.

Print information available on the last page.

ISBN: 978-1-4269-0505-6 (sc)
ISBN: 978-1-4269-0507-0 (e)

Trafford rev. 05/22/2019

Trafford PUBLISHING® www.trafford.com
North America & international
toll-free: 1 888 232 4444 (USA & Canada)
fax: 812 355 4082

Dedicated

To

Glenn & Anne

Foreword

The surgical treatment of weight loss has become more acceptable in the eight years since I began work on my first weight loss surgery book. Now, however, there are more options, and more information to review. At the time of writing, gastric bypass was the most common procedure performed in the United States for weight loss; there was good experience, and it was safe. Adjustable gastric banding was just starting to be used, and we did not have good information on how well it would work, how safe it would be, or how durable it would be. Now, we have seven years of experience with adjustable gastric banding and the body of information is excellent, and the numbers of patients choosing adjustable laparoscopic banding is increasing. But, there's a new operation that's available, and many are choosing to use that surgery to control their weight and to improve their comorbid conditions. The resolution of diabetes has been so successful for all three of these operations that we are now starting to consider surgery as a primary treatment of diabetes!

Since surgery has shown to be effective and safe, people are trying to get more information about their options. The Internet continues to be a major source of information for patients who want to improve their lives, but there is no way to be sure that what you read is accurate. This book is intended to help those patients obtain accurate information about weight loss surgery. This is a step-by-step manual of preparation that I require all of my patients to read.

Considering Weight Loss Surgery will explain in simple terms the way in which weight loss occurs, the methods available, and the methods that work. The current surgical options are presented, and there is a full review of the complications that may occur during or after surgery. It will explain what happens during surgery and how the surgery works. Most of all, it gives you the information you need to make a successful recovery from surgery, then a successful progression of weight loss.

My first edition was produced with the goal of creating an easy to read book that concentrates on the essential information needed to get you through the weight loss surgery experience. There was little information on postoperative menus and meal planning. There continue to be plenty of books and websites contributing to those subjects, but as my practice has developed, more materials for my patients has been gathered, and I have added these materials to this edition. Possibly the best place to get more information is the various support group meetings that are available in most cities. Here you will get to talk to patients who have already had surgery, and have developed strategies for becoming successful after surgery. I greatly encourage your attendance to these meetings.

It seems that people are realizing the effects of obesity on their lives and their families, and are more willing to consider surgery to treat this disease. However, the primary goal of surgery continues to be a change in the habits of eating. So surgery is a tool used to make adjustments in your eating habits. Remember, surgery does not cause weight loss, it causes behavioral changes in the way you eat. Only after making and maintaining those changes will weight loss occur and be sustained.

Like so many things in life, no one method works for everyone, and fortunately we now have multiple methods to help you make those changes. It remains up to the patients, with the guidance of their surgeon, to pick the tool that works best for them. But remember that screwdrivers make lousy hammers, and so the surgery you pick has to be used appropriately in order to successfully make the changes in your eating habits. If your eating habits do not change, you will not be successful in losing weight. The different surgeries have some things in common, but also significant differences, and it is important that you understand how your surgery works so that you can use it to obtain your best outcome.

It is also important to understand that weight loss is a balance of calories in, and calories out. Surgery can make remarkable changes in your ability to take calories in, but without appropriate calorie output, it remains difficult to lose an adequate amount of weight. Our bodies are designed to get a minimum number of calories in to be healthy, but if your calorie output falls below even this low level, then you cannot lose weight. It becomes a mathematical impossibility.

As our world has become less physical, more mental and more sedentary, we burn fewer and fewer calories day to day. So outside of the daily work we do, we must adopt an active lifestyle that includes a schedule of exercise for the sake of exercise. The mistake that most people make is in thinking that they have to kill themselves in order to get any exercise. The type of exercise I am talking about is as simple as walking four times a day, eight city blocks down and back. Or you can wear a pedometer at work to achieve 10,000 steps a day. Or you can use a light weightlifting program, an exercise video, or treadmill or other aerobic exercise for 30 minutes a day. You don't even have to exercise a straight 30 minutes at a time. You can break it up into as many segments as you need to help you achieve your exercise goal. It becomes important to choose an exercise that you like, on a schedule that you can complete. If you don't like it, you won't do it!

I know there is a lot of information to cover. My hope is that this book helps you to organize the information into a resource that you can keep with you, and that will help guide you, through the surgical experience and beyond.

Disclaimer

The practice of medicine is both science and art. The art is the ability to understand when the science starts and when it stops. Learning the art is a never-ending process.

For your best outcome, it is important that you take the advice of your personal physician to heart. Once you have committed yourself to surgery for weight loss, it is imperative that you allow your physician to lead you through the entire process until the course is clear. There is no substitute for the wisdom of your own physician, and although this book was created to help you smoothly negotiate the pathway of weight loss surgery, in no way is it to be used to argue with, undermine or take the place of your own physician or his/her advice.

Although my own experiences and education are the basis for the information contained in this book, information is always changing. I have tried to be as accurate as possible.

Acknowledgements

I want to thank my family for tolerating all the late nights at work, phone calls in the middle of the night, and the absences from family life that comes with being a surgeon. Also, I want to thank all of those who helped bring this book to fruition: Robert Robertson, who performed the copy-editing, to my colleague, Rajesh S. Padmanabhan, MD for his support, advice and friendship. A special thanks goes to my staff and team members: Kim Besancon, RN, BSN, CBN, who runs the program day to day, Lisa Badolato, RD, LD, our dietician and a contributer to the dietary section of this book, and Merrill Littleberry, LCWS, LCDC, CCM who keeps both ourselves and our patients sane.

Contents

Introduction

Imagine that you go to your doctor feeling tired all the time. You have become short of breath with the most minimal exertion and have pain in your hips, knees and back. Your ankles are swollen and it is difficult to walk. You may have serious life threatening diseases such as diabetes, hypertension, or sleep apnea. "Help me to feel better," you say to your doctor. "Save my life". Your doctor tells you that you have developed a serious disease called morbid obesity. This disease can lead to other diseases, disability, and early death. There are three basic treatments available.

The ideal treatment is a combination of reasonable calorie restriction, e.g., dieting and regular exercise. There are few risks, but unfortunately this approach seems to work for fewer than 5% of patients.

The next treatment involves medications to change your appetite or the way you absorb nutrients. Medicines can be added to diet and exercise, but do little to improve either the short term or long-term success. As new medications come out, more success may be seen, but there are also failures that have led to other health conditions for patients.

The final treatment involves surgery. Many will point out the increased risks associated with surgery. Certainly these need to be explored, but there is also a marked increase in the success of weight loss efforts with surgery. In the least successful surgeries, 40% of patients will lose and keep off over half of their excess weight. In the more successful treatments, 80% will lose and keep off 60 to 70% of their excess weight.

After explaining the options, your doctor then tells you that you need to choose a treatment, if you want to be treated at all. You realize that your options are limited. Morbid obesity is a life-threatening disease that induces other lifestyle limiting conditions. Diet and exercise are rarely successful. Is surgery the best choice for you? In this book I want to tell you why I think the surgery is the treatment to choose. I also want to guide you through the information you will need to make that choice.

Chapter One

Morbid Obesity Defined

The average weight in the United States is increasing by leaps and bounds. What makes this happen is a subject of speculation. It probably has something to do with the increase in fast-food meals, the high amounts of granulated or refined sugar in our meals, and a decrease in the daily activity of our population. Also, research recently suggested a genetic basis for obesity.

As recently as 100 years ago, it may have been rare for people in the United States to eat three square meals a day. Now we eat constantly. Until recently, daily living often required an output of 4000 or more calories per day. Now we get by with less than 2500 calories per day.

So our calorie intake has increased while our calorie output has decreased. This can be expressed in terms of the evolution of human society. Our social advances may have exceeded our body's ability to adapt. In the United States, we now produce much more calorie resource than the population needs to consume. We are animals designed to survive in a world of famine. Now that we live in a world of feast, we must ask ourselves, "Where is the balance that ensures a healthy life?"

To treat morbid obesity we need to know when weight gain becomes a problem and what its effects are. A standard way of measuring weight is needed, and each step up in weight has to be related to the risk of developing disease, the worsening of diseases already present, and the early loss of life due to diseases related to morbid obesity.

One method of measuring weight gain and its effects is to compare a person's height with his/her weight, and the illnesses that occur as weight increases. Currently obesity is defined by height versus weight measurements. Initially in 1983, researchers at the Metropolitan Life Insurance Company produced tables for height versus weight and correlated these measurements to how long their clients lived. Metropolitan Life sells life insurance policies; consequently it becomes important for them to know how long people live and why they die.

One of the things Metropolitan found in these comparisons is that people at certain heights live longer at a certain weight. As people get heavier, their life spans shorten in a directly proportional fashion. Initially the Metropolitan Life Insurance Company developed three sets of comparison tables. These were based on the size of the skeletal frame that patients presented. There was a table for small frames, a table for medium frames, and a table for large frames. For instance, if you had a small, slight frame, then it would not be fair to compare your weight to someone with very wide shoulders or hips, even if you stood at the same height. So three tables were developed.

Initially, morbid obesity was defined as 100 pounds over the weight listed in the 1983 Metropolitan Life Insurance Company tables. Although accurate, the three tables led to confusion because there was no standard way of determining who had a small, medium, or large frame. On the next page is the height and weight chart that doctors most often use.

Metropolitan Life Ideal Weight Chart			
Ideal Weight for Medium-Frame Men and Women			
Men		Women	
Height (inches)	Weight (pounds)	Height (inches)	Weight (pounds)
62	136	58	115
63	138	59	117
64	140	60	120
65	142	61	122
66	145	62	125
67	148	63	128
68	151	64	131
69	154	65	134
70	157	66	137
71	160	67	139
72	164	68	143
73	167	69	146
74	171	70	149
75	175	71	152
76	179	72	155
77	182	73	158
78	185	74	161

Because of this confusion, efforts were begun to create a single measurement. A measure called the Body Mass Index (BMI) was eventually developed to correlate with the Metropolitan Life Insurance Company tables.

The BMI is a calculation made by comparing height versus weight, much like the Metropolitan Life Insurance Company tables. However the BMI calculation uses measurements in the metric system. It compares weight in kilograms and height in meters. The formula is (weight in kilograms/ height in meters squared) or BMI = kg/m^2. If you want to calculate your own BMI, follow these steps:

Take your height in inches (twelve inches to a foot - five feet is 60 inches) and multiply it by 2.54 (the number of centimeters in an inch). This is your height in centimeters. For instance, a person five feet and six inches tall is 66 inches tall. Multiply that by 2.54 and that person is 167.64 centimeters tall.

Divide that number by 100. This is your height in meters. A person that is 167.64 centimeters tall is 1.6764 meters, or almost 1.68 meters tall.

Now, multiply your height in meters by itself: 1.68 X 1.68 = 2.82. This is the number that is on the bottom of the formula BMI = kg/m^2.

Next, convert your weight in pounds to your weight in kilograms. This is the top number in the formula BMI = kg/m^2. One pound is 2.2 kilograms. Take your weight in pounds and divide it by 2.2. For example, a 180 lb. person weighs 82 kg.

Take your weight in kilograms and divide it by your height in meters squared.

BMI = kg/m^2 = 82 / 2.82 = 29.

Now fill in your numbers

Height in inches _______ X 2.54 = ________ centimeters

Height in centimeters divided by 100.

________ / 100 = ________ meters tall

Height in meters multiplied by itself.

_______ X ______ = ________ meters squared

Weight in pounds divided by 2.2

________ / ________ = ________ kilograms

Formula for BMI = kg/m^2 _______ / ______ = ______ BMI

So what does your BMI tell you?

Overweight is a BMI of >27

Obese is a BMI >30

Morbidly Obese is a BMI > 40 and is called morbid because of the significant contribution to so many health conditions.

Body Mass Index Table

(Weight in Pounds X Height in Inches)

	55	**56**	**57**	**58**	**59**	**60**	**61**	**62**	**63**	**64**	**65**	**66**
100	23	22	22	21	20	20	19	18	18	17	17	16
110	26	25	24	23	22	21	21	20	20	19	18	18
120	28	27	26	26	24	23	23	22	21	21	20	19
130	30	29	28	27	26	25	25	24	23	22	22	21
140	33	31	30	29	28	27	26	26	25	24	23	23
150	35	34	32	31	30	29	28	27	27	26	25	24
160	37	36	35	33	32	31	30	29	28	27	27	26
170	40	38	37	36	34	33	32	31	30	29	28	27
180	42	40	39	38	36	35	34	33	32	31	30	29
190	44	43	41	40	38	37	36	35	34	33	32	31
200	46	45	43	42	40	39	38	37	35	34	33	32
210	49	47	45	44	42	41	40	38	37	36	35	34
220	51	49	48	46	44	43	42	40	39	38	37	36
230	53	52	50	48	46	45	43	42	41	39	38	37
240	56	54	52	50	48	47	45	44	43	41	40	39
250	58	56	53	52	50	49	47	46	44	43	42	40
260	60	58	56	54	53	51	49	48	46	45	43	42
270	63	61	58	56	55	53	51	49	48	46	45	44
280	65	63	61	59	57	55	53	51	50	48	47	45
290	67	65	63	61	59	57	55	53	51	50	48	47
300	70	67	65	63	61	59	57	55	53	51	50	48
310	72	70	67	65	63	61	59	57	55	53	52	50
320	74	72	69	67	65	62	60	59	57	55	53	52
330	77	74	71	69	67	64	62	60	58	57	55	53
340	79	76	74	71	69	66	64	62	60	58	57	55
350	81	78	76	73	71	68	66	64	62	60	58	56
360	84	81	78	75	73	70	68	66	64	62	60	58
370	86	83	80	77	75	72	70	68	66	64	62	60
380	88	85	82	79	77	74	72	70	67	65	63	61
390	91	87	84	82	79	76	74	71	69	67	65	63
400	93	90	87	84	81	78	76	73	71	69	67	65

Body Mass Index Table

(Weight in Pounds X Height in Inches)

	55	**56**	**57**	**58**	**59**	**60**	**61**	**62**	**63**	**64**	**65**	**66**
410	95	92	89	86	83	80	77	75	73	70	68	66
420	98	94	91	88	85	82	79	77	74	72	70	68
430	100	96	93	90	87	84	81	79	76	74	72	69
440	102	99	95	92	89	86	83	80	78	76	73	71
450	105	101	97	94	91	88	85	82	80	77	75	73
460	107	103	100	96	93	90	87	84	81	79	77	74
470	109	105	102	98	95	92	89	86	83	81	78	76
480	112	108	104	100	97	94	91	88	85	82	80	77
490	114	110	106	102	99	96	93	90	87	84	82	79
500	116	112	108	104	101	98	94	91	89	86	83	81
510	119	114	110	107	103	100	96	93	90	88	85	82
520	112	117	113	109	105	102	98	95	92	89	87	84
530	123	119	115	111	107	104	100	97	94	91	88	86
540	126	121	117	113	109	105	102	99	96	93	90	87
550	128	123	119	115	111	107	104	101	97	94	92	89
560	130	126	121	117	113	109	106	102	99	96	93	90
570	132	128	123	119	115	111	108	104	101	98	95	92
580	135	130	126	121	117	113	110	106	103	100	97	94
590	137	132	128	123	119	115	111	108	105	101	98	95
600	139	135	130	125	121	117	113	110	106	103	100	97

Body Mass Index Table

(Weight in Pounds X Height in Inches)

	67	**68**	**69**	**70**	**71**	**72**	**73**	**74**	**75**	**76**
100	16	15	15	14	14	14	13	13	12	12
110	17	17	16	16	15	15	15	14	14	13
120	19	18	18	17	17	16	16	15	15	15
130	20	20	19	19	18	18	17	17	16	16
140	22	21	21	20	20	19	18	18	17	17
150	23	23	22	22	21	20	20	19	19	18
160	25	24	24	23	22	22	21	21	20	19
170	27	26	25	24	24	23	22	22	21	21
180	28	27	27	26	25	24	24	23	22	22
190	30	29	28	27	26	26	25	24	24	23
200	31	30	30	29	28	27	26	26	25	24
210	33	32	31	30	29	28	28	27	26	26
220	34	33	32	32	31	30	29	28	27	27
230	36	35	34	33	32	31	30	30	29	28
240	38	36	35	34	33	33	32	31	30	29
250	39	38	37	36	35	34	33	32	31	30
260	41	40	38	37	36	35	34	33	32	32
270	42	41	40	39	38	37	36	35	34	33
280	44	43	41	40	39	38	37	36	35	34
290	45	44	43	42	40	39	38	37	36	35
300	47	46	44	43	42	41	40	39	37	37
310	49	47	46	44	43	42	41	40	39	38
320	50	49	47	46	45	43	42	41	40	39
330	52	50	49	47	46	45	44	42	41	40
340	53	52	50	49	47	46	45	44	42	41
350	55	53	52	50	49	47	46	45	44	43
360	56	55	53	52	50	49	47	46	45	44
370	58	56	55	53	52	50	49	48	46	45
380	60	58	56	55	53	52	50	49	47	46
390	61	59	58	56	54	53	51	50	49	47
400	63	61	59	57	56	54	53	51	50	49

Body Mass Index Table

(Weight in Pounds X Height in Inches)

	67	**68**	**69**	**70**	**71**	**72**	**73**	**74**	**75**	**76**
410	64	62	61	59	57	56	54	53	51	50
420	66	64	62	60	59	57	55	54	52	51
430	67	65	63	62	60	58	57	55	54	52
440	69	67	65	63	61	60	58	56	55	54
450	70	68	66	65	63	61	59	58	56	55
460	72	70	68	66	64	62	61	59	57	56
470	74	71	69	67	66	64	62	60	59	57
480	75	73	71	69	67	65	63	62	60	58
490	77	75	72	70	68	66	65	63	61	60
500	78	76	74	72	70	68	66	64	62	61
510	80	78	75	73	71	69	67	65	64	62
520	81	79	77	75	73	71	69	67	65	63
530	83	81	78	76	74	72	70	68	66	65
540	85	82	80	77	75	73	71	69	67	66
550	86	84	81	79	77	75	73	71	69	67
560	88	85	83	80	78	76	74	72	70	68
570	89	87	84	82	79	77	75	73	71	69
580	91	88	86	83	81	79	77	74	72	69
590	92	90	87	85	82	80	78	76	74	72
600	94	91	89	86	84	81	79	77	75	71

Chapter Two

Why Treat Morbid Obesity?

It seems like an easy question to answer. Why do we need to even worry about being overweight? Many people try to convince you that the only reason weight loss is important is to avoid the peer pressure to conform to the ideals of what society thinks is acceptable. The pressure to "look good" and to be "desirable" can be intense. I do not think these are good reasons to be concerned about your weight. You should be happy with who you are and how you live your life.

But beware! There are many out there who will tell you that you should feel good about your size no matter how much you weigh. They say that the body knows how heavy you should be and you should not fight it. There are support groups, books, and celebrities that will help you feel better about yourself if you are overweight. But they are leading you astray. Your doctor knows that the more overweight you become, the worse your health is. Your health is why you should lose weight.

Even though it is important to have a good self image, and to feel like you are not some spectacle to be stared at or made fun of, a voice inside you tells you that something is not right about weighing so much. It is a voice you should pay attention to. Being overweight means more than looking different than others, it means your health is at risk. This is the true reason you should be concerned about your weight.

You may have health conditions but not even realize it. The most common complaints of the morbidly obese are shortness of breath with little or no exertion, getting tired very easily or early in the day, back pains and joint pains are common, as are painful varicose veins and swelling of the ankles, feet, and hands. Other complaints include heartburn, losing urine when coughing or sneezing, and irregular menstruation in women. These are signals from your body that you are hurting yourself. You may think that these problems are a normal part of life, and that you need to learn to put up with them. Nothing could be further from the truth.

Shortness of breath and early fatigue are signs that your body size has overwhelmed the ability of your heart and lungs to adequately function for you. Back pains and joint pains are signs your body's framework has reached its structural limits. Swelling of the hands, feet, and ankles are signs that the pumping action of the heart is no longer sufficient for the new miles of arteries and veins. Heartburn and leaking urine are signs that the valves designed to keep fluids in their appropriate compartments are overwhelmed. The increased pressure that the extra weight is exerting overwhelms the seal these valves provide. A history of irregular periods is just one sign that the hormone systems of the body are out of sync. These are conditions that many do not consider significant enough to treat aggressively, but which can make life miserable. These are also conditions that can be dramatically improved with weight loss.

Conditions like high blood pressure, diabetes, congestive heart failure, high cholesterol, arthritis and others are conditions that everyone recognizes as life threatening, clearly lead to more suffering, more disease, and early death. How common are these conditions in the morbidly obese? They are very common. Hypertension is seen in up to 60% of the patients. Diabetes is seen in up to a third. Lung dysfunction, which can lead to heart failure, is almost always present when your BMI reaches 60. Elevated fat and cholesterol levels in the blood contribute to the early death that is seen in any patient with morbid obesity. As a matter of fact, an incremental increase in weight is directly proportional to an incremental decrease in lifespan.

The ultimate test of a medical treatment is whether it decreases the number of patient deaths from disease. If your BMI is 40, your risk of death is over 250 times the normal risk. If your BMI is 50, your risk of death is more than 1000 times the normal risk. If a patient undergoes weight loss to a BMI less than 30, it does more to prolong their life than having a heart bypass surgery.

In terms of money, the cost to you as a patient is enormous. Each year $30 billion dollars is spent in commercial weight loss programs. The problem with spending this money is that none of these commercial weight loss programs have more than an almost accidental occurrence of significant long-term weight loss. In addition, each year $45 billion dollars in direct medical care costs is incurred. A large portion of that money comes from the Medicare and Medicaid budgets. The increased cost of treating the illnesses related to morbid obesity is a huge drain on our nation's resources. It takes money away from research for the cures to other illnesses. It takes money away from our schools and police and firefighters. It takes money away from our infrastructure. This is money that can be used for other needs if we take an aggressive approach to treating morbid obesity. In the private sector, morbid obesity is estimated to cost society $140 billion. These are the costs associated with missed work, poor production, support of the disabled, and so forth.

So the reasons for treating morbid obesity are clear. Living at a weight that is appropriate for your height will allow you to live a longer and healthier life. Undergoing surgery to lose weight allows you to lose the weight without wasting your money.

In the history of medicine and mankind, many different methods of controlling weight were attempted - herbs and brews, pills and procedures. Some of these treatments seem like they should have been obvious and immediate successes. For instance, wiring the mouth shut used to be a recommended procedure for weight loss. Seems simple that if you wire your mouth shut you won't eat much and automatically lose weight, right? Those patients not only did not lose weight, but also developed nutritional deficiencies. They learned to eat the wrong things in the wrong way to get around the wiring.

Other herbal solutions were not so clear as to how they cause you to lose weight, but still have fantastic claims of weight loss. Often they have testimonials from people who have lost weight. But they never tell you the total number of people taking the pills and the total number of those people who have successfully lost the weight. Just as importantly, they do not tell you how many of the people who are taking their pills developed other serious medical problems from taking those pills.

There are thousands of weight loss programs and diet plans advertised on television and radio. There are similarly thousands of books for sale in the bookstores giving advice on weight loss. How many of their readers have lost a significant amount of weight and kept it off? How successful have their diet plans been?

It is important for patients to know what is out there, and how successful or unsuccessful those treatments are. It is very important to know what else can happen to you if you take those herbal remedies, or participate in diets that radically change what you eat, or the mix of foods you eat. You cannot make an informed choice about what you are willing to try without this information. If the salespersons pushing these programs and pills on you do not know these answers, then you must seriously question the success and safety of these methods. That is the beauty of medicine in the United States. The regulations may be cumbersome in getting some medicines and treatments to the patients, but when they are offered, good information is available to you concerning the successes, the risks and the outcomes associated with the products and proposed procedures.

Chapter Three

The Goals of Weight Loss Therapy

Whenever we discuss weight loss with patients we make it clear that surgery is not the only answer. In fact, surgery is the last resort. For many, the challenge of losing weight is like trying to move a ten ton boulder. It stands in the middle of the road to success and is much too heavy to move. There is no going around the rock in our way.

When you consider weight loss therapy, though, you have to give the patient a pickaxe, send them to the nearest edge of the rock and let them pick away at it. It takes a long time, but eventually, with the right tools, they will turn the boulder into a pile of pebbles that can be moved out of the way. We have to give our patients the resources to make small changes a little bit at a time in order to be successful in the long run.

Sounds great, huh! So how do we do that? Where do I get those tools? The first thing to do is to start out with goals or objectives that are achievable. This is the problem with very low calorie diets. Placing the body on a calorie intake of less than 1000 calories per day is stressful to the body. You develop cravings and often depression. The body does not have the raw resources to take care of the basic maintenance needs from day to day. Patients fail because eating only 1000 calories a day is an unobtainable goal. A reasonable goal for calorie intake is probably 1800 calories per day. It's usually less than you will burn in a day, so you will see weight loss, but not so low that you get physiological rebellion from the body.

Now, in order to lose weight, your calorie output has to be larger than your calorie intake. In other words, your activity level has to be enough to burn, say, 2500 calories per day. Exercise physiologists say that you need at least 300 calories in exercise output per day to be healthy. So exercise becomes a necessary tool to add to the toolbox.

So now we have some goals for weight loss. About 1800 calories per day of intake, and about 2500 calories per day of output, which includes an exercise program of 300 calories per day. This will be effective to lose weight without going out of your mind because of hunger. If you have lost weight and are at a stable level, then your intake and output will be equal. Extra intake means you will gain weight, and extra output means you will lose weight.

Calorie output

How do we take this information and make it usable for the patient? Well, the output part is easy. Develop an exercise program that you can do five out of the seven days a week. This will vary for each patient, because some people like walking, some like treadmills, some dance, some ride horses or bikes. It doesn't matter so much what you do, so long as you like it. If you hate it, you probably won't do it for very long.

Your exercise regimen should be aerobic, meaning when you exercise you should not be short of breath. It's okay to get your heart rate up moderately, let's say to a pulse rate of 110 to 120 beats per minute. We now need to breakdown our exercise goal into something we can measure.

One of the very important concepts that patients need to understand about weight loss is the need for measurement. We need to measure both intake of calories and output of calories. It's very important to have the measurement because that's the only way that we can be assured of moving towards and eventually reaching our goals. Measurements provide the frame of reference to let us know where we are. If you are in the middle of the ocean with no landmarks, it's tough to tell whether all the paddling you are doing is getting you anywhere. In the same way, measurements are the landmarks we use to make progress. It's the only way that we can be encouraged by our progress, and discouraged by our lack of progress. Then these emotions have to be channeled into a successful change. Many patients say to me "I move around a lot at work, so that's my exercise every day". I have to ask them, "Well, how much exercise is that?" No one knows because it's not measured. So the first thing to do is what we call *structured exercise*. That means exercising just for the sake of exercising, in a structured way that allows an accurate measurement of calorie output.

Exercise Regimens

In order to exercise 300 calories per day, do at least one of the following:

Walk 4 miles per day

10,000 steps per day

30 minutes of aerobic exercise a day

When we exercise, it's good to know that you don't have to do all that exercise at once. When you haven't been exercising regularly, you also have to develop a level of basic fitness that has been missing, so you won't want to start at these goals, but work up to them.

If you want to walk for exercise, start out with four scheduled walking trips per day. First thing in the morning, before or after lunch, before or after dinner, and at night before you turn on the evening news. You can start out by just walking 50 yards out then back. Again, measuring the distance is important so that you know you have achieved your goal. Each week double the distance you walked the week before, so that at the end of six weeks, you are walking about half a mile out then half a mile back four times a day. That's four miles a day, and now you've reached your goal.

If you want to use weights, a very easy regimen is an upper extremity program. Most of us are weaker than we should be in the shoulders and arms, so this is a good program for everyone. Plus, those with back and hip and knee problems can do these easily.

Start by buying some 3 lb weights. There are four exercises in this program.

1. Arm curls
2. Forward arm extensions
3. Sideways arm extensions
4. The overhead military press.

Begin by doing three reps of each of these exercises four times a day. Increase by three reps each week until you are doing twelve reps of each exercise four times a day. Then you can increase the number of sets you do each time you stop to exercise. Your goal is to do four sets a day, so you can do two sets in the morning and two in the evening, or just do all four at once when you first get up. Then you can hop into the shower and get your day started.

If you are super-busy and don't feel like you can stop to exercise, then wear a pedometer. You can measure how much unstructured exercise you get each day by looking at how many steps you walk a day. If it's less than 10,000 steps per day, you will need to add some exercise in somewhere in the day. Park farther away in the parking lot. Use the stairs instead of the elevator. Do whatever you can to increase the number of steps you walk a day. Most often you will be making small adjustments in your day-to-day routine to improve your calorie output.

Calorie intake

Now how do we take the 1800 calorie a day goal and make it useable? Well, most people eat three times a day. So instead of thinking of a daily goal, let's think of a meal goal of 600 calories per meal. It's very easy to look at the nutritional information and tell if what you are eating for that particular meal is going to exceed the 600-calorie limit. Maybe you are hungry all day long, and it's hard not to snack between meals. Then change to eating six times a day, but limit the meals to 300 calories per meal. This is fairly easy to keep track of as well.

One of the requirements for a healthy diet is to get enough protein in per day. Protein promotes muscle growth, and most of our calorie output is due to muscle activity. So the more muscle you carry around the more calories you burn around the clock. If you are hungry between meals, protein intake is very filling and may improve the hunger pangs you have. I suggest using protein drinks, especially if you are on the six meals per day program. Two or three of those meals can be substituted with a protein drink. Now, there are a lot of different protein drinks out there, and some are advertised as protein drinks, but don't have that much protein, and contain a lot of calories. So your goal for the protein drink is at least 25 grams of protein per serving, and less than 300 calories per serving. Now you are fulfilling several goals at once:

adequate protein intake, a meal that satisfies your hunger, and avoiding excess calorie intake.

It's also important to realize that we are not talking about dieting here. We are trying to create a healthy lifestyle of eating that has so far escaped you. Many people diet during the week, then celebrate their successes on the weekend. That's a recipe for failure, and I will show you why.

Lets say you eat 2000 calories a day for the first five days of the week, and achieve a calorie output of 2500 calories per day using your exercise regimen of 300 calories per day. That's pretty good success during the week. You are still losing 500 calories per day, and at the end of the week that will equal about a pound of weight loss. If you keep that up all month you've lost four pounds. If you keep that up all year, that's fifty pounds.

So let's say you decide to celebrate. You've done a good job, so its time to reward yourself. You go out with friends for dinner, you serve up some ice cream, or you order out a pizza. It's extremely easy, especially in the eating environment we live in today, to get in 4500 to 6000 calories in one day. So what is your calorie balance for Saturday? Well, you burned your 2500 calories, but you ate 5000 calories. That means you are 2500 calories behind for the weekend and you've completely wiped out your progress for the week. This is why "dieting" is all wrong and why people rarely make a successful attempt at weight loss. Instead of developing a lifestyle, in which they wake up each morning with the same eating plan as they always have, they are only making temporary changes that they don't intend to keep over the long run.

Why do people fail to lose weight or regain weight that they have lost? Three basic elements exist in weight gain.

First, eating large volumes of food with normal calorie density. Second, eating normal volumes of high calorie foods. Third, eating normal amounts of normal density food but maintaining an inadequate calorie output. Each factor by itself, or in combination with the others prevents weight loss or will cause weight regain. It's a routine of eating moderate amounts of a normal calorie density diet in a setting of regular exercise that defines the healthy lifestyle.

So to summarize our goals:

We need some form of exercise that equals 300 kcal per day by walking four miles per day, walking 10,000 steps per day using a pedometer, or 30 minutes of aerobic activity per day.

We need to maintain an intake of 600 calories per meal in a three meal day or 300 calories per meal in a six meal day.

We also need protein intake to support muscle growth, up to 100 grams per day.

This book will give you lists of foods and their calorie and protein content. In addition, there are several internet sources to create diet diaries with. Diet diaries are very effective in helping patients track their calorie and protein intake. I recommend www.fitday.com

Chapter Four

Medical Treatment of Morbid Obesity

Although the main purpose of this book is to tell you about the surgical treatment of morbid obesity, it is important to know that there are medical treatments. Medical treatments should always be tried before surgical treatments. Unfortunately, one of the first things to note about medicines for the treatment of morbid obesity is that they are not very successful. Some medicines were taken off the shelf because of the unacceptable medical risks that occur when these medicines are taken. Of the remaining medicines, the amount of weight lost is not significant enough to warrant the costs of the medicines. Of the scientific data we have to compare (instead of the common commercial testimonials) most of the studies involve short-term results, from ten weeks to a year in length, and the average weight loss is only about 30 lbs. (15 kg). How much money will you spend on a medicine that only helps you to lose 30 lbs.? In addition, if you quit taking the medication, you will more than likely gain the weight back, plus some extra.

The 1992 National Institutes of Health's (NIH) study of obesity showed that about 95% of morbidly obese people fail to lose and keep off an acceptable amount of weight with medical therapy and exercise. Perhaps this is a reflection of how hard it is to change 20 or 30 or more years of eating and exercise habits. It helps to review this information, however, so that you know what options are available and the relative success of any other treatments.

You should always try diet and exercise before taking medications, and you should always try medical therapies before surgical therapies. It is not worth going through the risk of surgery if a medicine can take care of the problem. Sometimes, though, the surgical cure is so much better than the medical cure that it becomes the preferred method of treatment. A good example is the treatment of gallstones.

For years different non-surgical methods for curing gallstones were tried. We found that some stones can be crushed with sound waves sent through a tub of water. Unfortunately gallstones are created in several different chemical combinations, and only a small minority of them breakup with sound waves. It becomes too expensive to build and keep that kind of equipment available for so few people.

Medicines were also developed to help the body dissolve gallstones. Patients must take these medications two to four times a day for six months to a year, and when they stop taking the medicines the stones often develop again. The medicine is very expensive and tastes extremely bad, so a lot of people never take the medicine once it is prescribed.

Eventually they form gallstones again or get an infection of the gallbladder that comes back over and over again because of the stones. Surgery removes the gallbladder so that stones can no longer form. The gallbladder concentrates the bile that the liver produces for the breakdown and absorption of fatty foods. Once the gallbladder is removed, the bile flows into the bowels without being concentrated, but still works well to break down and absorb fatty foods. Since surgery works, is relatively safe, and prevents the problem from recurring, it became favored over the medical treatment for gallstones. The medicines for obesity underwent the same kind of evolution, and currently surgery is the favored treatment for obesity.

There are three main medical therapies in conventional medicine right now. Most are designed to change the way that your brain tells you that you are hungry. The hope for these medications is that people will not overeat if they are not hungry. The problem is that people eat for all kinds of reasons besides being hungry. They may be nervous, depressed, or just bored. The other problem is that it is very hard to lose weight without also increasing your level of exercise. Just taking medicine to lose weight does not address this necessity. There are also medications that act to increase the number of calories that your body burns by increasing your metabolism. Most of those medications were found to have unacceptable or sometimes dangerous side effects.

Sibutramine is the generic name of the medicine marketed as Meridia®, which acts as an appetite suppressant. A yearlong trial of 485 patients showed up to 14 lbs. (6.1 kg) weight loss, but there are side effects of an increased heart rate and blood pressure. It is one of the more commonly prescribed weight loss medications.

Other medications were designed to block the body's ability to absorb what you eat. That sounds great! You can eat whatever you want without having to count calories or anything! The problem is that some of the vitamins and fats that are necessary for good health are also blocked by these medications.

Orlistat is the generic name of a medication marketed as both Alli® and as Xenical®. It suppresses an enzyme called pancreatic lipase. This is an enzyme that breaks down fat into small particles that your body can absorb. Orlistat blocks up to 30% of your ingested fat calories. A one-year study showed weight loss of around 23 lbs. (10.3 Kg) in 343 patients. However, most regained their weight after coming off the medication. Side effects are mostly due to fat passing through to the stool giving oily stools, soft stools, or diarrhea. The other problem is that when patients want to eat a tasty, fatty meal without the side effects, they just stop taking the medication.

Phentermine is the third and most successful drug. It is the Phen of Phen-fen. Phen-fen was taken off the market in September of 1997, due to an increase in leakage across the heart valves. This was felt to lead to heart failure in some patients and was also blamed for the deaths of some patients. When Phentermine was studied alone, it did not lead to these side effects or deaths. In a study of 108 patients over nine months, patients had an average weight loss of 27 lbs. (12.2 kg). Interestingly, when compared to the Phen-fen combination, Phentermine alone caused more weight loss alone than in combination. Patients lost an average of 25 lbs. on Phentermine vs. 20 lbs. on Phen-fen (11.3kg vs. 9.3kg).

Although all of these drugs are shown to lead to weight loss, they seem to be limited both in degree and duration. Patients who stop taking these medications regain their weight, and often put on more weight. In patients who are morbidly obese, losing only 25 lbs. is nowhere near enough weight loss to affect the illnesses associated with morbid obesity.

Chapter Five

Surgical Treatment of Morbid Obesity

In comparison to medical treatments, surgical treatments are found to be fairly successful in treating morbid obesity, with anywhere from 40% to 70% or more of excess weight loss. In 1992, the National Institutes of Health (NIH) came out with a consensus statement. Part of that statement was that surgery is a therapy that may be offered to those who met the criteria of morbid obesity and failed medical therapy for weight loss.

Like medical therapies, multiple surgical therapies are available, and although in 1992 the NIH only recommended two of them, we now have four operations available. They are called laparoscopic adjustable banded gastroplasty (LABG), vertical sleeve gastrectomy (VSG), roux en Y gastric exclusion (RY-GE or RNY), and bilopancreatic bypass with duodenal switch (BPDS). There have been other operations available, but these are the current procedures. And all of these operations are basically divided into three categories: restrictive procedures–limits the volume of food one can take in at one sitting; malabsorptive procedures–limits the body's ability to absorb what you are eating; mixed procedures–which use both restrictive and malabsorptive effects. Traditionally the mixed procedures are shown to have the better weight loss of the malabsorptive procedures while fewer of the complications of malnutrition like the restrictive procedures. But each operation has specific changes in your eating habits, so you must also consider which operation works best for you.

Restrictive Procedures

Restrictive procedures, and the restrictive part of mixed procedures, work in two ways. First, the procedure limits the amount of food you can eat at one setting. Pouch procedures, like the laparoscopic adjustable gastric band procedure, create a pouch out of the top of the stomach to limit food volume. Other examples include the silastic ring vertical gastroplasty, horizontal banded gastroplasty, and the vertical banded gastroplasty. The newest procedure, laparoscopic sleeve gastrectomy, creates a narrow tube out of the stomach to limit volume.

Importantly, all procedures with a restrictive component also produce a second mechanism of calorie restriction called satiety. Satiety means that once you eat, you do not get hungry again immediately. Satiety occurs because the outlet to the new pouch is very small, so the food empties the pouch very slowly. Many patients say they are only hungry in the morning, then remain satisfied the rest of the day. This is a very important mechanism because even if you only eat a little bit at a time, if you are still hungry you will continue to eat all day long. This will still allow enough calorie intake to prevent weight loss. So it's important to eat small meals three to six times per day, remain satisfied after a meal for three to six hours, and avoid grazing on foods between meals.

Malabsorptive Procedures

Malabsorptive procedures limit what your body can absorb by bypassing the majority of your small intestine. The ileo-jejunal bypass was the original malabsorptive procedure, but was abandoned due to episodes of malnutrition, liver failure, and an elevated number of deaths. It was later modified to more successful forms. The duodenal switch and the biliopancreatic bypass are two of the more common malabsorptive procedures. Only about two feet of small bowel is used to absorb food once it is mixed with the digestive enzymes. Most surgeons now combine the two surgeries into a single procedure called biliopancreatic bypass with duodenal switch.

Mixed Procedures

The Roux en Y gastric bypass is the most common of the mixed procedures. The top of the stomach is divided to create a small pouch that limits the volume of food you can eat at a meal. A portion of the small intestine is then connected to the pouch to move food past the lower portion of the stomach. The outlet from the small upper pouch to the intestine is made to a small size to slow the progress of food out of the pouch, which creates satiety. The food is delivered to the lower portion of small intestine, where the food is allowed to mix with the digestive enzymes. The use of some of the small intestine to bypass the lower portion of the stomach prevents it from being used to absorb food. Typically six feet or more of small intestine is still available to absorb food, so the effect is not as drastic as with the purely malabsorptive procedures.

The Roux en Y gastric bypass does have a fourth method of action to help maintain the patient's weight loss. It is a side effect of bypassing the outlet control of the stomach and is called the "dumping" syndrome. When patients who have this operation eat foods high in fat content, or high in the content of simple sugars, they immediately get ill. When the small intestine is exposed to high concentrations of fat and simple sugars the patient feels weak, nauseated, dizzy, sweaty, and often get abdominal cramps or diarrhea. Because it happens immediately, these patients learn to avoid the foods that contain fats and simple sugars. These are foods that are high in calories but very small in volume. These are the foods that continue to allow patients to consume a high number of calories despite the volume restriction that is present after surgery. When patients are able to make a change in this eating behavior it may be the factor most responsible for the long-term success of weight loss surgery. Patients learn that it requires a change in the way that they think about eating. The surgery produces a behavioral modification. Then you have to learn to choose your foods wisely.

Explaining the Different Surgical Options

All three types of surgical procedures are used today in the treatment of morbid obesity. Your surgeon may have strong opinions as to which technique is best for you. This often depends on how much excess weight you need to lose, why your doctor feels you have gained the weight in the first place, and to some extent on the procedure your doctor feels most comfortable performing. You should also have some say about which procedure is performed, and you need to know more about these surgeries before you can make an intelligent decision.

Restrictive Procedures

Restrictive procedures are designed to work in two major ways. The first effect is produced by partitioning the stomach into a small pouch. The small pouch will limit the volume of food that a person can eat at one sitting. If the patient eats more than the pouch holds, then they vomit up the excess food. Since, in general, people don't like to vomit every time they have eaten;

they tend to avoid overfilling the pouch. Various techniques are used to teach patients to eat small bites, to chew very thoroughly, and to eat slowly. These techniques help patients to avoid vomiting when they eat, and create a change in the behavior of eating. They no longer eat so fast that they over eat at every meal, and they no longer eat large meals. They also learn to eat frequently to avoid getting too hungry.

The second effect is called early satiety. This means that when patients eat a meal, they feel full and stay full for a long period of time. Patients are not hungry even when they only eat a small meal. This occurs because the outlet to the small pouch is made to be very narrow. It's like having a small cup with a small hole in it. If you fill the cup with water, the water empties very slowly. With soft or solid food, it may take 3 or 4 hours to empty the pouch, so patients feel full until the pouch empties.

These procedures have undergone significant changes over the past twenty to thirty years as physicians have learned more about how the body and patients respond to the volume restriction. New procedures, like the adjustable gastric band or the gastric sleeve operation, have decreased the complexity and possible complications associated with these surgeries.

Horizontal and Vertical Gastroplasty

Although these techniques are no longer favored, they are important procedures in the development of all the other procedures now in use today. The stomach is partitioned with staplers to allow a small pouch for food to be initially deposited in. The outlet from the pouch was controlled by how close the stapling came to the edge of the stomach. The horizontal gastroplasty showed early failure rates due to two problems, stretching of the dome of the pouch and dilation of the outlet of the pouch.

Horizontal banded gastroplasty

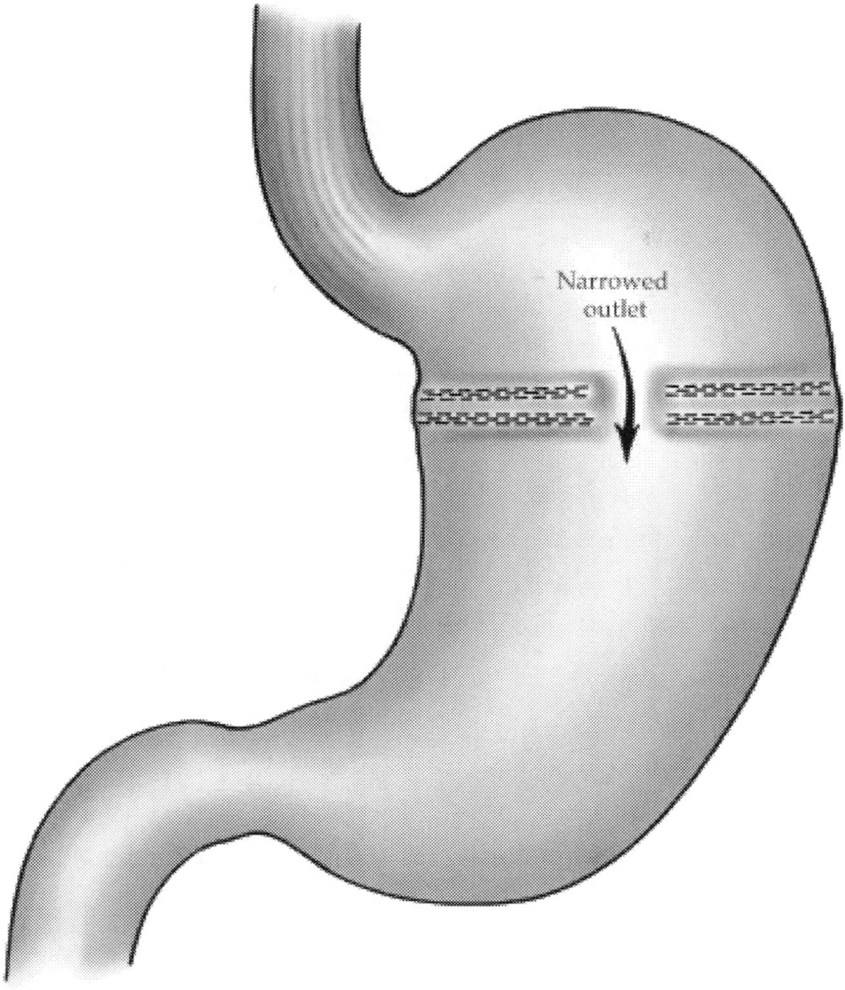

To address these problems, the vertical gastroplasty was developed. The terms horizontal and vertical refer to the direction of the staple line on the stomach. So the application of the staples changed from a horizontal orientation to a vertical orientation.

Vertical banded gastroplasty

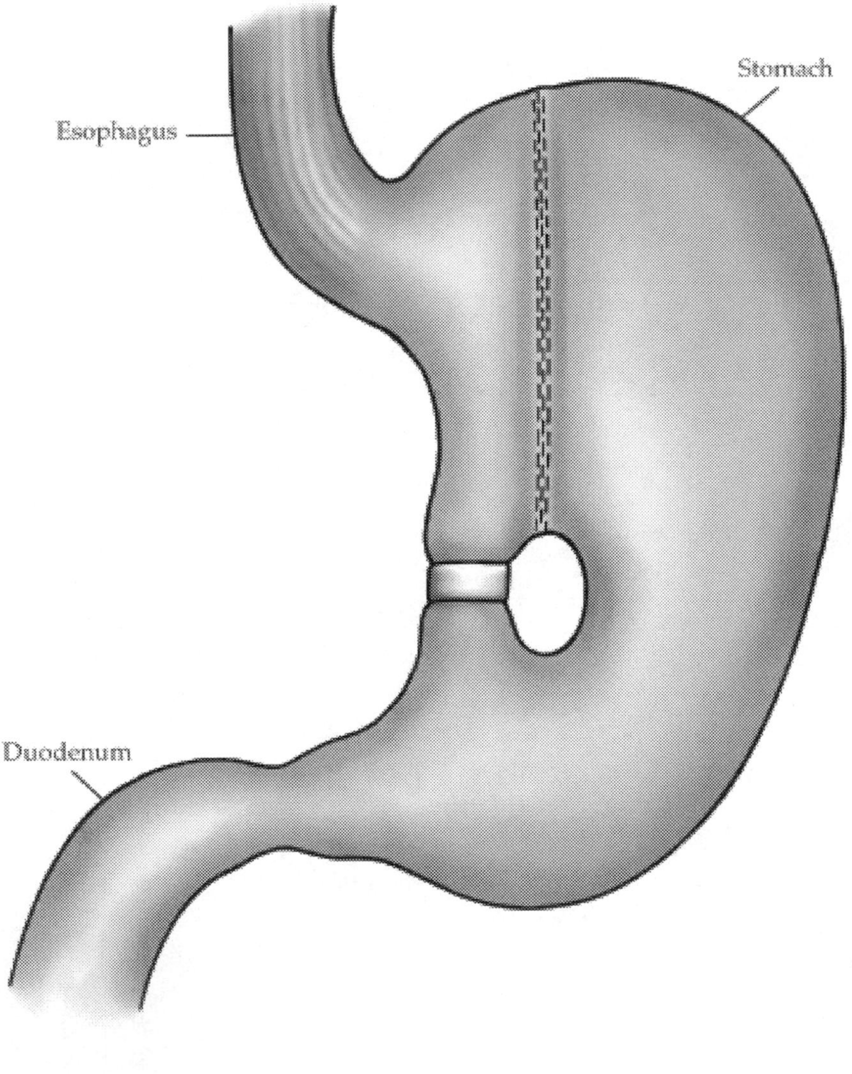

The outlet of the pouch would still dilate though, and let the pouch empty quickly, so a silastic ring was added to the pouch outlet to keep it from dilating. Eventually the silastic ring vertical gastroplasty fell out of favor because the artificial material began to erode into the stomach or the staple line would fail, allowing food to pass into the larger stomach portion, ruining the effect of volume restriction and prolonged satiety. In general, neither of these techniques is used any longer.

Laparoscopic Adjustable Gastric Banding

The adjustable laparoscopic band technique has been used in Europe for many years and was introduced into the United States in 2001. Since that time it has become very popular and we now have good studies on its outcomes.

Laparoscopic adjustable gastric band

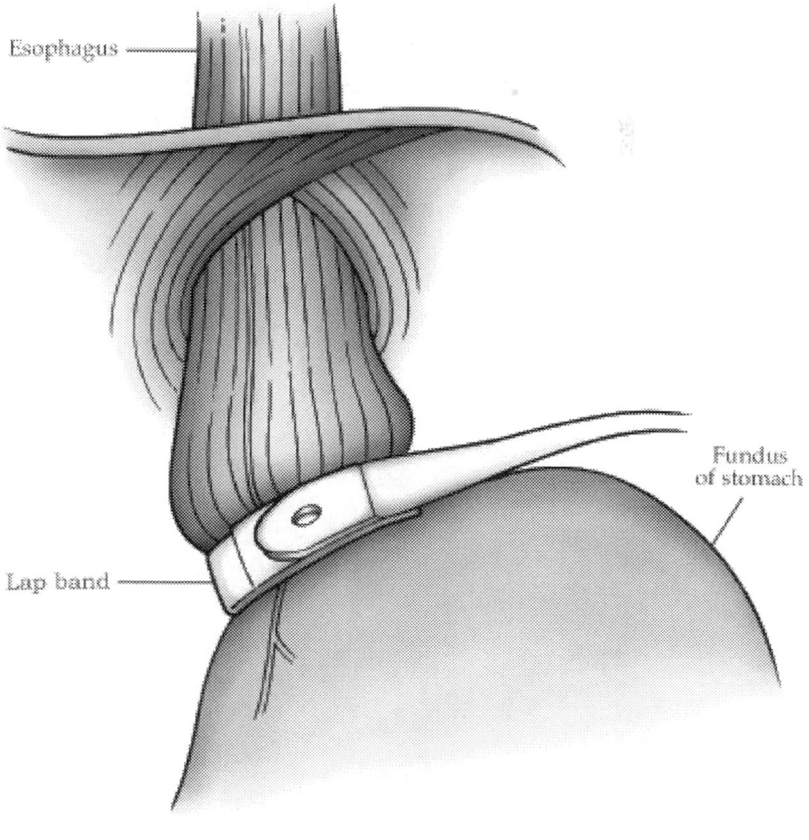

In this operation, the top of the stomach is gathered into a pouch that holds about half a cup. A soft plastic tubing with an inner cushion is used to keep the pouch gathered. The pouch itself limits the amount of food that you can eat at one sitting. The outlet of the pouch is controlled by the cushion, which can be inflated to decrease the outlet size, or deflated to increase the outlet size. Outlet size determines satiety.

The goal is to inflate the band enough to allow food to pass slowly out of the pouch which prolongs satiety. Since patients are not hungry, they don't eat as often. As patients lose weight, the cushion is adjusted to minimize their level of hunger. The fact that the band is adjustable is a major reason for its popularity, but it also means that reliable, regular follow-ups with your surgeon are absolutely essential for your success. In addition, the fact that it can be easily removed is often felt to be an advantage for this technique, but the patients have a tendency to regain their weight once the mechanism of their weight loss has been removed.

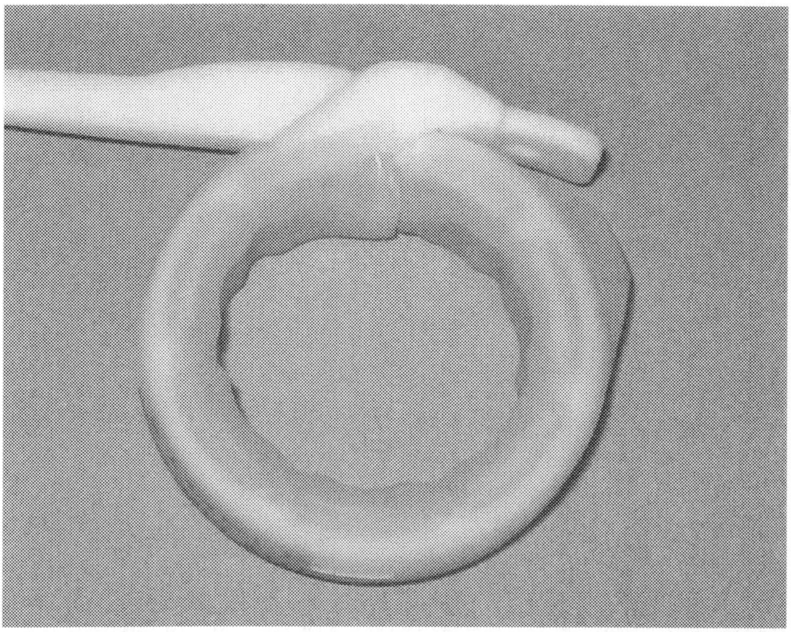

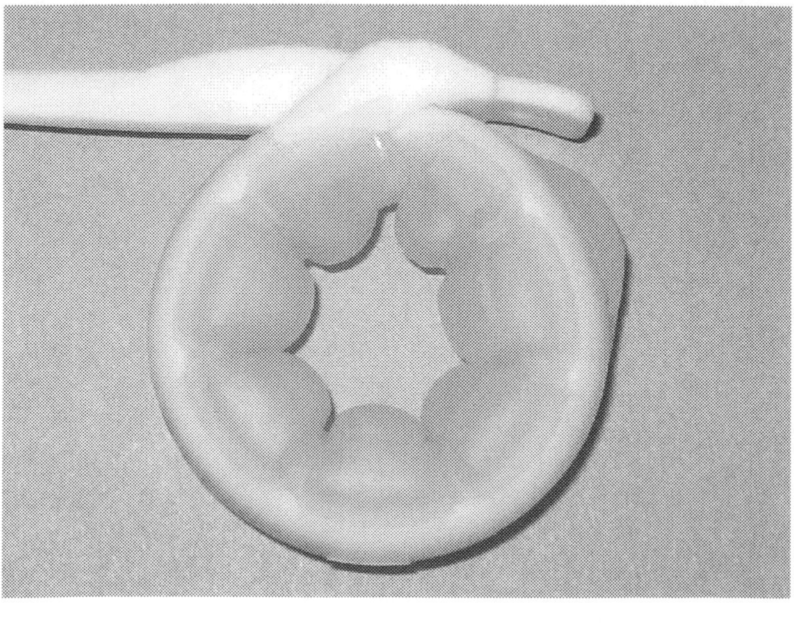

Laparoscopic Vertical Sleeve Gastrectomy

The laparoscopic vertical sleeve gastrectomy started out as part of the biliopancreatic bypass with duodenal switch procedure. These procedures produce the greatest weight loss but also the most complications. In very high risk patients it was decided to try staging their operations to decrease the risk of surgery. So one part of the surgery would be performed and the patients would lose some weight, making the second part of the procedure easier to perform. What surgeons found was that the first part of the procedure produced such good weight loss in some of the patients, that they didn't need the second part of the procedure. So it was decided to try the first part of the procedure by itself as a weight loss technique. That first part is called a vertical sleeve gastrectomy.

In a laparoscopic vertical sleeve gastrectomy operation, the majority of the stomach is stapled off and removed from the body, leaving a long narrow tube between the esophagus and the small bowel. The original procedure actually left a fairly large tube, but by narrowing the tube, better weight loss is achieved. This occurs because the narrower tube allows volume restriction, only small meals can be eaten. It also produces satiety because the narrow tube slows the passage of food out of the stomach.

The laparoscopic vertical sleeve gastrectomy produces better weight loss than the laparoscopic adjustable gastric band, but introduces some of the more serious complications because cutting of the stomach is required. It has only been used in the United States as a stand-alone procedure since about 2005, so the operations durability and long term effects are still being studied. It is also the only weight loss surgery that is truly non-reversible.

Laparoscopic sleeve gastrectomy

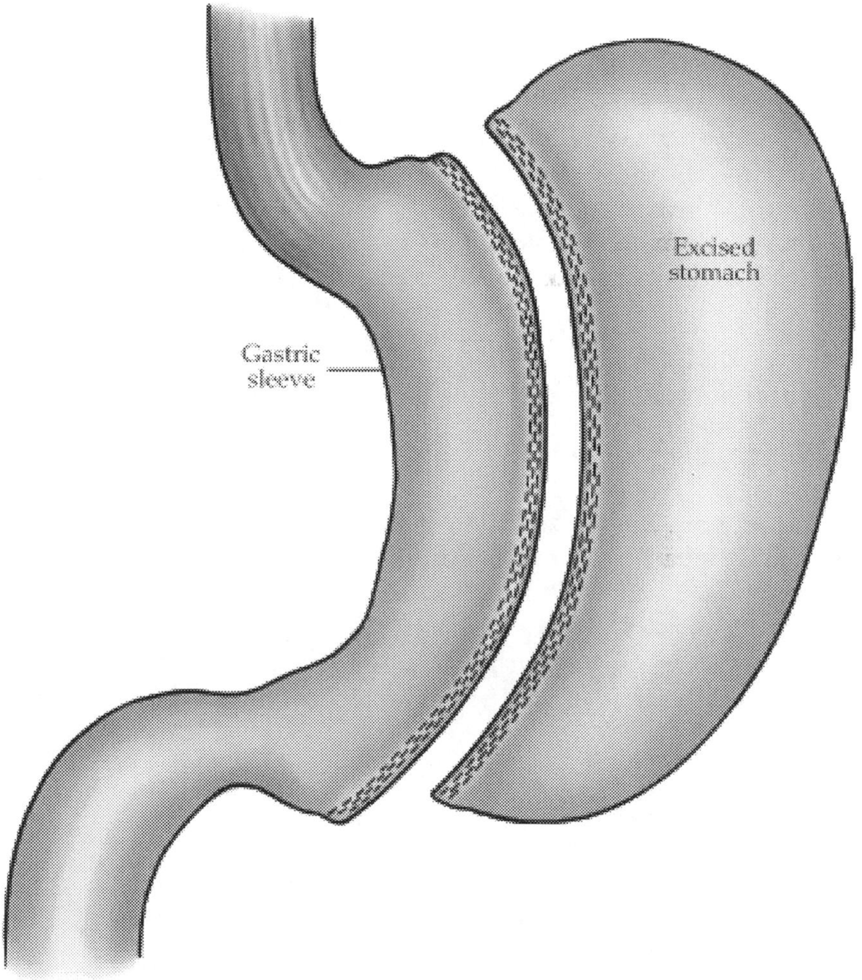

The benefit of the restrictive procedures is that they are technically the easiest weight-loss surgeries to perform. Although there is suturing of the stomach and in the case of the vertical sleeve there is cutting of the stomach, there is no cutting and sewing of the small bowel, and no bypass of the small bowel, so little protein or vitamin deficiency occurs.

The problems of the restrictive procedures include less overall weight loss and possibly a tendency to regain weight. The outlet of the pouch can get blocked or obstructed. "Sweet eaters" are patients who crave and eat a lot of sweets, and can cheat by eating simple sugars all the time. They eat a high number of calories in very small volumes. When prosthetic materials are used to create the small pouch, erosion of prosthetic materials through the stomach wall can occur. With the laparoscopic adjustable gastric bands, the port site used to inflate the band can have its own set of complications.

Malabsorptive Procedures

The second major type of procedure is called a malabsorptive procedure. These procedures cut and bypass the small bowel to limit your body's ability to absorb what you eat. The ileo-jejunal bypass was the original malabsorptive procedure. It bypassed almost the entire small bowel. However the procedure was abandoned due to a high occurrence of malnutrition, liver failure and an elevated death rate. These problems are not seen in the newer techniques of small bowel bypass.

Biliopancreatic Bypass with Duodenal Switch Procedures

The biliopancreatic bypass with duodenal switch is now a single procedure, but it began as two procedures that worked by keeping the enzymes needed for digestion from the food that is taken in. The enzymes produced by your body must break down food into the small components that are absorbed. After this surgery, food enters the stomach and passes into the small bowel, but the digestive enzymes are diverted to the end of the small bowel. Before enzymes are added, absorption is difficult because the molecules are too large. After this type of bypass, only about two feet of small bowel is available to absorb food once the food is mixed in with these enzymes. After the enzymes are added, the food is broken down to small molecules, but very little is absorbed in this short distance.

The benefit of this surgery is that it works consistently. Patients have shown sustained loss of about 70% to 90% of their excess weight, and the amount of bypass is adjustable to a patient's size. However, the problems can be severe. Malabsorption can also lead to nutritional deficiencies, especially of proteins and vitamins. It is more difficult to estimate how much bowel to bypass before bringing the enzymes and food together. Like the ileo-jejunjal bypass, daily episodes of fatty stools and diarrhea are not uncommon for patients. Because of the risk of major malnutrition and micronutrient malabsorption, routine follow-up is a must for these patients, both in the short term and in the long term.

Biliopancreatic Diversion with Duodenal Switch

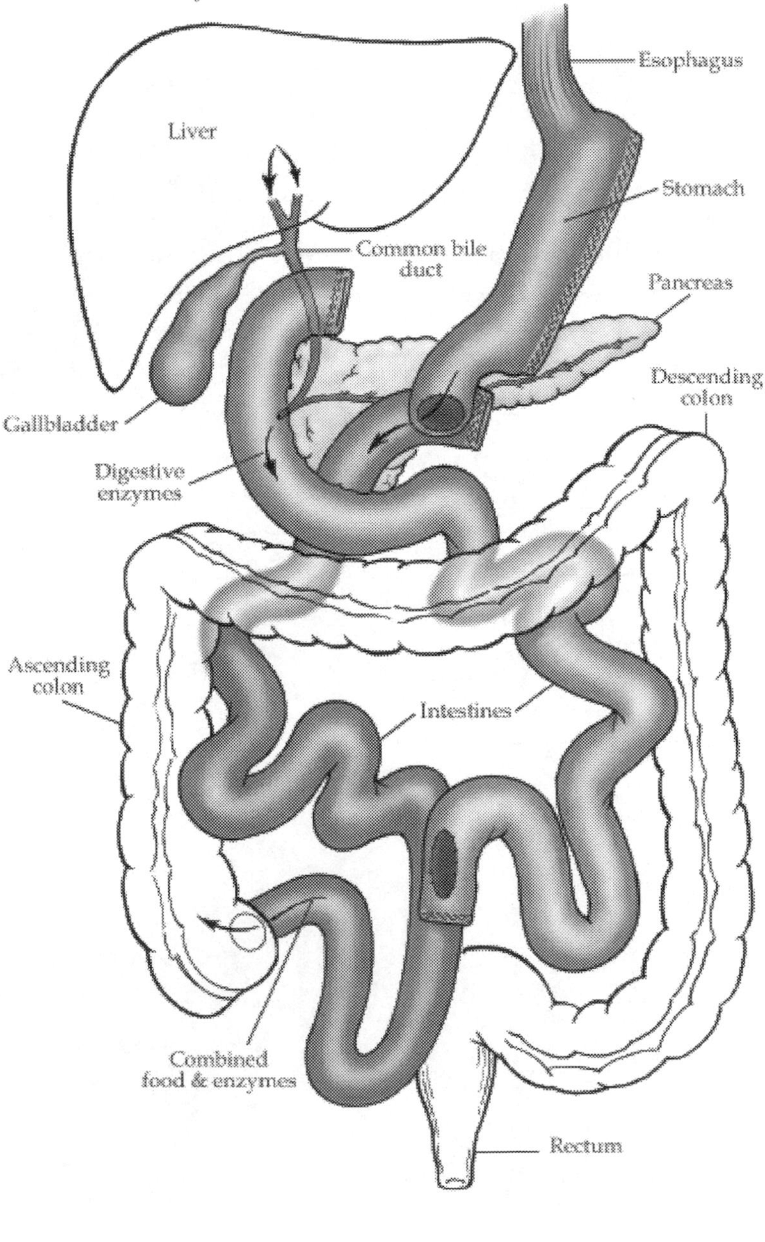

Mixed Procedures

The recognized problem of the restrictive procedures is that patients can eat small amounts of high calorie foods by eating simple sugars and fatty or fried foods, thereby getting enough calories to prevent weight loss. The problem with malabsorptive procedures is that so much of the small bowel is bypassed that nutritional deficiencies develop. If a shorter length of bowel is bypassed, then patients are able to take in enough volume of food to prevent weight loss. That is why a mixed procedure was developed, to take the best of the restrictive and malabsorptive procedures, while minimizing the bad side effects of each.

Roux en Y Gastric Bypass (RY-GE or RNY)

The most common weight loss procedure performed today is a mixed procedure. It is called the Roux en Y Gastric Bypass. In the past it was performed almost exclusively as an open operation. Now it is performed almost exclusively as a laparoscopic operation. It combines cutting the stomach to create a small pouch and bypassing the rest of the stomach with a short length of small bowel. The connection of the pouch to the small bowel is made to a certain size to allow food to pass slowly out of the pouch, producing prolonged satiety.

The enzymes for digestion produced in the lower stomach portion are diverted for a short segment to join the small bowel that was connected to the pouch. Once the food moves out of the pouch, the connected small bowel transports the food into the portion of bowel that the digestive enzymes have moved into. The food and the enzymes mix, the food breaks down to smaller molecules, which then allows us to absorb our food. This part of the small bowel, called the common channel, is usually at least four times as long as the malabsorptive procedures.

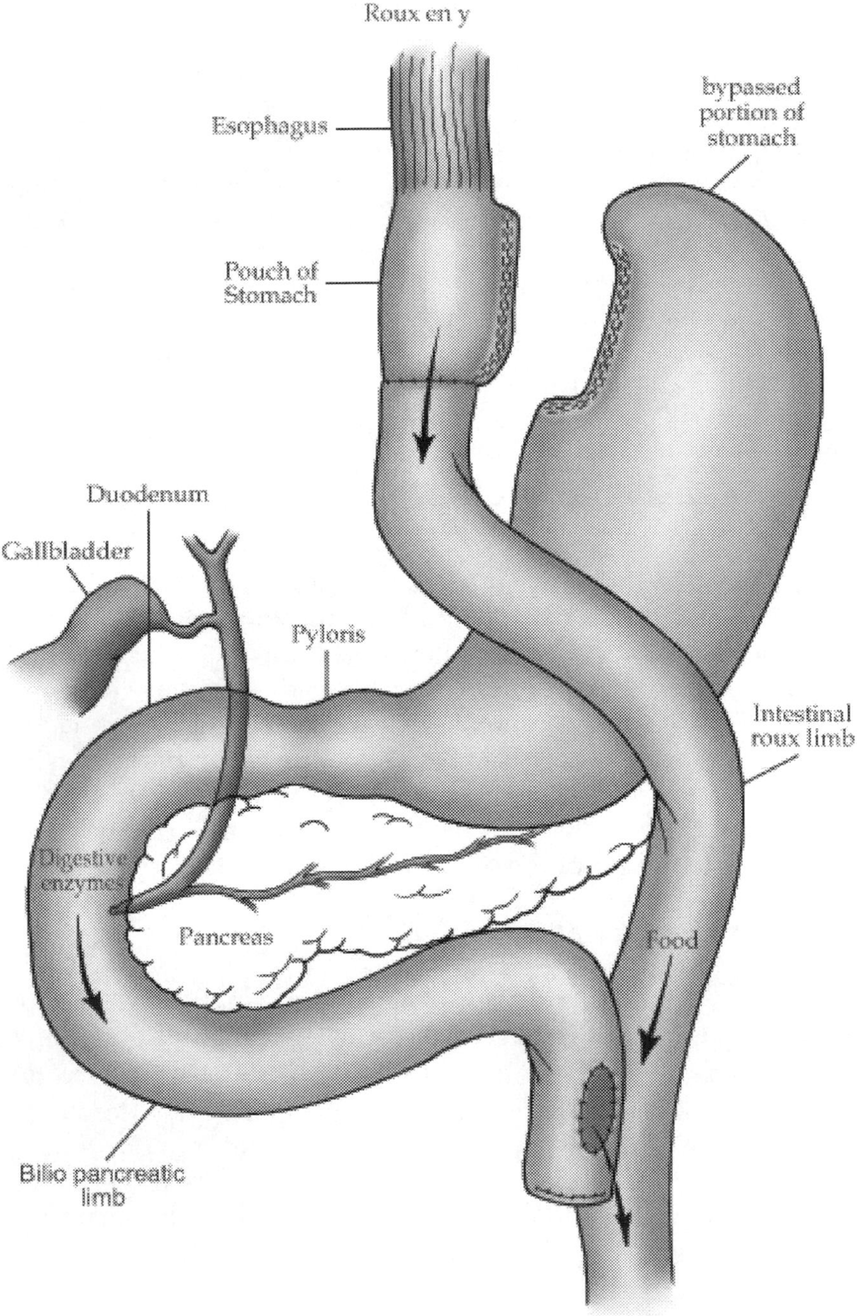
Roux en y
Esophagus
bypassed portion of stomach
Pouch of Stomach
Duodenum
Gallbladder
Pyloris
Intestinal roux limb
Digestive enzymes
Pancreas
Food
Bilio pancreatic limb

There are four main reasons for patients losing weight after this surgery. First, the small pouch restricts the volume of food you can eat at one setting, so no more large meals. Most patients eat six small meals per day. Obstruction, or food getting stuck in the pouch, occurs much less than with the banding procedures. This may be due to the lack of plastic banding material, as natural tissue may give more flexibility to the outlet of the stomach pouch.

The second reason patients lose weight is satiety. Their hunger cravings are curbed. This is because the outlet of the pouch is made to a certain size that prevents rapid emptying of the pouch, so patients stay full for longer periods of time. Patients are less likely to "graze" during the day if they don't feel hungry.

The third component of weight loss is malabsorption. When food and digestive enzymes are mixed in the small bowel, foods are broken down to small particles that are absorbed through the wall of the small bowel for use by the body. In gastric bypass operations, the small bowel is used to bypass the lower stomach. This portion of bowel receives food from the pouch, but there are no enzymes, so absorption of food is poor in this segment of small bowel. Similarly, the portion of small bowel coming from the lower stomach contains enzymes, but not food, so no absorption occurs there. It's not until the food and enzymes mix in the common channel that nutrients can start to be absorbed. So creation of the "Y" bypass induces some malabsorption. However this may not be a major mechanism of weight loss, since there is plenty of intestine in the common channel, and studies of the small bowel suggest that, with time, the bowel will become more efficient at absorbing calories after bypass.

The fourth component is called the "dumping" syndrome. This component has two effects: intolerance to concentrated sweets, and intolerance to high fat foods.

The first effect is caused by bypassing the first part of the small bowel, which causes nausea, sweating, weak knees, and a generalized ill feeling if the patients eat refined or granulated sugar in any form, e.g., baked, sprinkled, glazes, or sauces. Concentrated sweets like molasses, honey, and corn syrup can also cause "dumping." The more complex sugars, like the ones found in fruits and vegetables usually do not cause "dumping." Since most people do not eat things that make them sick, they learn to avoid these sweets.

The second effect is an intolerance to fatty or fried foods, which causes abdominal cramps, nausea, and diarrhea. Anything fried or cooked in oil, any of the high fat meats like prime rib, bacon, or ham, can cause these symptoms. Again, patients learn to avoid these foods because they cause them to get sick.

There are many surgeons who see the dumping syndrome as an unwanted side effect, or a complication of the gastric bypass operation. Instead, I think that this procedure is unique in using the "dumping" syndrome as a benefit. The side effect of the "dumping" discourages the patient from two major sources of increased calorie intake, e.g., simple sugars, and high fat foods. Patients experience "dumping" soon after the food is eaten, and they learn to relate the bad experience with those foods. This causes a change in the way patients behave, and the way they think about eating. I think this behavior modification is most responsible for the long-term success of this procedure. Patients have been shown to maintain weight loss for over 20-year periods of time.

Patients should know that there are potential problems with this surgery, too. It is a more technically challenging surgery than the restrictive procedures because the small bowel is cut and sewn twice. Vitamin deficiencies do occur, but are less common and less severe than with the malabsorptive procedures. The most common vitamin deficiencies are iron, calcium, B12 and folate.

These nutrients can be replaced using over-the-counter vitamins and do not require a prescription or a visit to the doctor to get started on them. The trade off for all the hypertension, diabetes, cardiac, arthritis and reflux medicines is probably well worth it.

Chapter Six

Considering Surgery for Weight Loss

To some extent, you put your life at risk when going to surgery so it is important to understand what those risks are. Just as importantly, patients who are morbidly obese also must understand that their weight is putting their lives at risk as well. So how do you relate those two sets of risk.

When I talk to my patients, I relate surgery to driving down the highway. Every day you get into the car and drive 70 mph down the highway. As you go down the highway, you almost always see cars on the side of the road or in the ditch. Sometimes they are just broken down, but often you see a car damaged in some sort of accident. When you see this, you know that people crash and die on the highway every day, but you still get in your car and drive down the highway. You don't really know what the risk is. You don't know how many people crash each day, or how many miles are driven before a crash occurs, but you have been driving for a while and in your head you calculate some sort of risk. When you do, you decide that getting where you are going and doing what you need to do is worth the risk of driving.

You also know that there are things you can do to minimize the risk. You can drive on good tires that are properly inflated. You can avoid debris in the road. If another driver seems reckless, you can pull away from him/her. You can avoid drinking and driving. You follow the advice of road signs. All these things help make your trip to the grocery store safer. In the same way, your surgeon's preoperative and postoperative program will give you the information you need to make surgery safe for you.

So, the first decision you have to make concerns what you want surgery to do for you. What are you trying to achieve? Is it just weight loss? Is it controlling diabetes or hypertension? Is it to get pregnant?

Weight loss surgery can treat many different disease processes. They include: Diabetes, hypertension, hyperlipidemia, early heart disease, asthma, sleep apnea, pulmonary hypertension, congestive heart failure, swelling of the legs, varicose veins, reflux disease, stress urinary incontinence, osteoarthritis, degenerative joint disease, menstrual irregularity, infertility, and several cancers. The number of disease processes, and their severity, will change both the risk of surgery and the benefit of surgery.

Because the different surgeries have different mechanisms of action and different outcomes, it's important to know what your goals are. Is achieving that goal worth the risk of surgery? Which surgery is best for achieving that goal?

Comparing the different surgeries:

In this chapter we will compare the three major surgeries used for weight loss in the United States today: gastric banding, gastric sleeve, and gastric bypass. In fact, these surgeries have a lot in common, but they also differ significantly in terms of weight lost and their success in treating comorbid conditions.

First lets review the similarities. All three surgeries can be performed laparoscopically. Usually, five small incisions are used to perform each surgery. Although the hospital stay can differ, these same incisions take the same amount of time to heal, so the recovery is practically the same for each surgery. The preoperative preparation is likely to be the same for all three surgeries, and the postoperative recovery diet is the same. Initially starting with liquids for the first three weeks, then pureed foods, soft foods and finally back to solid foods by the sixth postoperative week. This gives the surgery time to heal on the inside.

All three surgeries rely on regular patient follow-up to achieve success. For gastric banding patients, adjustments to the band are crucial for success. If you don't get your band adjusted, it just doesn't work, and you will not lose weight. For gastric bypass patients, it is particularly important to follow lab work in the first year, so that vitamin and mineral deficiencies are monitored and treated. Along with gastric bypass, gastric sleeve patients need careful follow-up of their lab work, meal volumes and food tolerances.

Complication rates are also similar among the three surgeries, although the types of complications can vary. Although reports in the literature can vary significantly, I think that a fair average is about a 15% non-fatal complication rate. A full review of risks is undertaken in following chapters, but each surgery has its own set of risks that are more likely to occur. For instance, gastric sleeves tend to have more nausea and food intolerances. Gastric bands tend to have more problems with the band becoming infected, leaking or moving. Gastric bypass patients have more vitamin deficiencies. All of these problems are treatable, but are also time consuming and aggravating for both the surgeon and the patient.

The rate of fatal complications is similar, but not the same. For gastric bands and gastric sleeves, mortality rates are around 0.1%. For gastric bypass, the mortality rate is closer to 0.5%. At first glance, it seems that gastric bypass is 5 times more fatal than bands or sleeves, and that is statistically correct. But is it clinically relevant? In other words, if you have to operate on a thousand patients to see a difference in mortality rate, then how much does that weigh in on your decision of which surgery to choose?

The real differences in the surgeries include differences in weight loss, how fast you lose weight, and the rate of resolution of major comorbid disease processes. There are also differences in hospital stays.

The Band

The laparoscopic gastric band is mostly performed as an outpatient procedure. You come in, have surgery, and go home the same day.

The average weight loss at one year is 30% of excess weight. The average weight loss at two years is 40% of excess weight, and at three years about 50% of excess weight. Most literature reports put the weight loss maintained long term at 40 to 50 percent excess weight loss. Some series report 50 to 70% excess weight loss with follow up every 6 weeks for three years. There is a failure rate of approximately 30%, where the band is removed due to failure to lose at least 25% of excess weight, or a complication requires removal of the band and conversion to a gastric sleeve or gastric bypass. The weight loss outcome is almost completely dependent on the patient's follow-up for band adjustments. Many patients will achieve better weight loss, but a similar number of patients will have very poor weight loss. Additionally, since the band is a restrictive procedure only, patients have to avoid the low volume high calorie foods on their own. Unfortunately, there is no mechanism to punish you for eating french fries and ice cream sundaes nor is there one to prevent you from doing so, but if you do that enough, even in small volumes, you will not lose weight.

The laparoscopic adjustable gastric band is effective at treating most of the major comorbid conditions. However differences exist with resolution of both diabetes and hypertension. In diabetics, an analysis of several studies shows about a 48% incidence of resolution of diabetes. With hypertension, approximately 38% of patients get off of their medications.

Patients choose the band because they perceive it to be safer than the operations that include cutting or stapling. The diet is more flexible than gastric bypass in terms of eating sugars and fats and it is the easiest surgery to reverse or to convert to another procedure.

The Sleeve

The laparoscopic vertical sleeve gastrectomy is performed laparoscopically, but because it's a relatively new procedure, patients are staying in the hospital two to three days. There seems to be more episodes of nausea and vomiting, which have to be controlled with IV medications before the patient can go home.

The laparoscopic vertical sleeve gastrectomy has no long term data, but short term information is promising. Early results indicate about a 60% loss of excess weight by 18 months after operation. Importantly, this is the only non-reversible surgery that is currently being performed for weight loss. Similar to the band, the sleeve relies on volume restriction and prolonged satiety to help keep patients from eating too much or too often. But it also has the same problem with high calorie low volume foods, there is no mechanism to keep patients from sipping on milk shakes all day. So patients have to be compliant with avoiding those foods.

Early results from sleeve studies report approximately 60% resolution in diabetes and in high blood pressure. Weight loss from any of these surgeries results in improvement of most of the other conditions related to morbid obesity. These include asthma, sleep apnea, osteoarthritis, degenerative joint disease, stress urinary incontinence, infertility and menstrual irregularity.

Patients should avoid choosing the sleeve if they have reflux (heartburn) or a history of ulcers in the stomach. Patients choose the sleeve over the other operations because it doesn't require adjustments for success. Some patients just don't want a foreign body (the band) implanted. Patients with persistent anemia or those who wouldn't tolerate any malabsorption are better candidates for a sleeve. Patients who have malabsorptive diseases such as ulcerative colitis or Crohn's disease may be better treated with a sleeve. If you have severe osteoarthritis and are requiring the use of non-steroidal anti-inflammatory drugs (NSAIDS), the sleeve allows you to continue taking those medications, which are generally discouraged in band and bypass patients.

Differences exist in the size of sleeve that is recommended. We use a sizing device to make the sleeve a certain diameter. If it becomes too small in diameter then more nausea and vomiting occur. If the healing process creates a thick scar along the sleeve, it may have to be converted to a gastric bypass operation. If the sleeve is too wide, then restriction and satiety are not as good, and there may be less weight loss. We do know that the sleeve dilates with time, and may need an operation in the future to re-size the sleeve or to convert it to gastric bypass. There is no long term data to suggest what the overall failure rate will be with the gastric sleeve, but we do know that some patients will either regain weight or not lose enough weight initially.

The laparoscopic roux en Y gastric bypass

Laparoscopic gastric bypass can be performed with the same five small incisions as the other two surgeries. The hospital stay is usually overnight, but can sometimes require a two night stay.

Patients lose weight on a fairly predictable schedule:

6 weeks.......................10 to 15 % excess weight loss

3 months.................... 20 to 25% excess weight loss

6 months.................... 40% of excess weight

9 months.................... 50% of their excess weight

One year.......................60 to 65% of their excess weight

18 months.................. 80% of excess weight

This weight loss schedule is almost completely dependent on the amount of exercise a patient does each week. For example, a patient who never exercises will almost never lose more than 50% of excess weight, even at two years after the operation. A patient who exercises for thirty minutes twice a week will most likely achieve a maximum of 60% excess weight loss. For patients that exercise for thirty minutes at least 4 times a week, 80% excess weight loss is common.

Most patients lose the maximum amount of weight at 18 months, and then can regain some weight, especially if they slip back into bad eating habits or reduce their exercise schedule. The gastric bypass is best known for the "dumping syndrome". Many consider this an unwanted side effect of the surgery, but it becomes a major reason why patients lose more weight. Patients with a "restriction only" operation have been known to adapt to poorer eating habits. Instead of eating 6 small meals of solid foods a day, they begin to drink high-calorie liquids. By substituting these high calorie sources for solid food, they are able to maintain a high daily calorie intake, and fail to lose weight. In contrast, gastric bypass patients tend to avoid these foods because of the dumping syndrome. Because surgery bypasses the lower stomach, with its hormone and control mechanisms, simple surgars cause you to feel ill. Eating simple sugars like store bought sugar, the corn syrup food manufacturers add to so many foods, honey or molasses, causes nausea, cramping, sweats, shakiness, rapid heart rate, dizziness and lightheadedness. These effects occur within 30 minutes of eating refined sugar, and the symptoms will last two to three hours. Similarly, fried foods or foods high in fat cause nausea, cramps and diarrhea.

Because these effects occur in close relation to eating certain foods, patients tend to avoid those foods, or even develop an aversion reaction to those foods. Since these are all high calorie, low volume foods, the total calorie intake from day to day tends to be less for gastric bypass patients, so they tend to lose more weight.

Patients who must take NSAIDS or have malabsorptive diseases, should not choose gastric bypass. Patients who perceive that gastric bypass is more dangerous will choose one of the other surgeries.

Patients who decide to have gastric bypass choose this operation because it has been used for weight loss in the United States since the 1960's, and so has a long history of safety and efficacy. The risk of death after surgery is less than the risk of death for some of the more common surgeries done in the United States, such as gallbladder surgery.

The weight loss for gastric bypass is clearly superior than the other two surgeries, and the resolution of diabetes and hypertension is much higher. A meta-analysis report of several thousand patients shows that 84% of diabetics get off of their diabetes medications altogether. The longer you have had diabetes, the less successful the operation is at allowing you to get off all the medications, but you will at least reduce your total medication use. So a patient whose blood sugars are uncontrolled on 100 units of insulin will often get complete control on just 10 units of insulin.

The improvement in diabetes is so remarkable, that studies have been undertaken outside the United States to treat diabetes primarily with surgery. These studies have shown significant success, so much so that Medicare is now considering whether to allow surgery as a covered benefit for the treatment of diabetes alone, without any weight criteria at all.

For patients with high blood pressure, approximately 75% will get off their medications. Again, the longer you have had high blood pressure, the less likely you will be to get off of all the medications, but your overall medication doses will likely decrease. All of the other comorbid conditions discussed earlier have high rates of improvement as well.

Chapter Seven

Consultation Information for Weight Loss Surgery

In order to understand how surgery creates weight loss for patients, and in order to understand the risks involved, patients need to have a long sit-down consultation with their surgeon of choice. Many patients make an appointment to see their surgeon about the weight loss surgery, and they already know a lot of the information needed to make a decision about whether or not to have the surgery. However many patients have not looked up the information, and rely on their surgeon to give them a complete set of information at the initial consultation. The initial consultation should provide the patients with all the information they need to make an informed choice, but there is a lot of information to sort through, and this chapter serves to organize some of that information and remind the patient of the surgeon's important points.

Why Surgical Patients Lose Weight

It is important to realize that patients lose weight after surgery because they change the way they are eating. The surgery does not cause them to lose weight. Surgery forces them to change the way they are eating. Eating differently will reduce the number of calories eaten each day.

Some will say that surgery creates an abnormal way of eating but I think that patients who are morbidly obese are eating abnormally already. They are consuming an abnormal number of calories each day. Surgery creates a situation in which they are able to change their eating habits to eat a normal number of calories each day.

Each of the surgeries listed in this book have different mechanisms of weight loss, but the eating habits that need to be formed are the same no matter which surgery you are having. Unless you eat healthy, you are going to gain weight, one way or the other. By healthy eating, we mean eating six small meals a day to obtain a calorie intake between 1200 and 2500 Kcal per day. The calorie intake varies some depending on your level of daily activity. You will also need to ensure an adequate protein intake, usually requiring 60 to 100 grams per day. Incumbent in the healthy lifestyle is an exercise program that includes 300 kcal of aerobic exercise a day.

People eat a large number of calories in different ways. Some will just eat a large volume of food. Others will mostly eat sweets. Many eat out a lot, and eat a high proportion of fried or fatty foods. Most people use a combination of these to eat a large number of calories.

Many people will eat healthy all week, then binge eat on the weekend, wiping out any progress they made during the week. People eat because they are anxious, nervous, bored, depressed, unhappy, or a variety of other reasons. The continuous nature of their eating leads to a large calorie intake. In any case, the large number of calories has to be continuously eaten day after day to maintain weight.

Losing weight is all about the math. The number of calories you eat minus the number of calories you burn. You have to expend a greater number of calories than you take in to lose weight. Most people burn 1200 to 1800 calories per day without exercising. If they are eating 1200 to 1800 calories, they will have a stable, healthy weight.

Calorie Intake	Calorie Output	Weight
1800	1800	Stable

If the calorie intake increases and the output stays the same, then weight increases.

Calorie Intake	Calorie Output	Weight
1800	1800	Stable at 150 lbs.
4000	1800	Gain to 250 lbs. (+2200calories/day)

In this example, there are 2200 extra calories. Not all of these calories may be absorbed and converted to weight gain. This may explain the genetic basis for differences in weight gain. Some people will gain all 2200 calories in weight and some will gain only part of it.

As you gain weight, you have more tissue to support, and so more calories are used to support the tissue. You have to carry the extra weight, which is just like exercising with a backpack full of weight. You have to feed the extra tissue every day, just like you have to eat to maintain the rest of your body. Most importantly, you have to keep warm. Keeping that extra tissue at 98.6 degrees Fahrenheit takes a lot of extra calories. When you weigh enough to use up all the calories you are taking in, then your weight stabilizes again.

Calorie Intake	Calorie Output	Weight
1800	1800	Stable at 150 lbs.
4000	1800(+2200calories/day)	Gain to 250 lbs.
4000	4000(increase due to weight gain)	Stable at 250 lbs.

The goal of surgery is to regulate a patient's ability to intake a healthy number of calories each day. When this occurs, then patients start to lose weight. As they lose weight, they burn fewer calories and start to lose weight at a slower rate.

Calorie Intake	Calorie Output	Weight
1800	1800	Stable at 150 lbs.
4000	1800	Gain to 250 lbs. (+2200calories/day)
4000	4000	Stable at 250 lbs.
1800	4000	Lose 10 lbs. per month at 250 lbs. (-2200calories/day)
1800	3000	Lose 5 lbs. per month at 200 lbs. (-1200calories/day)
1800	1800	Stable at 150 lbs.

Of course you can increase your calorie output by exercising. Exercise allows you to control how fast and how much weight you lose. You may also gain some weight back when you decrease or stop your exercise.

One of the big problems with recommending exercise is that most patients start out trying to exercise too hard and too fast. They get discouraged easily and quit before seeing any results. I tell my patients to first obtain a baseline of fitness by using a graduated walking program or a graduated upper extremity weight program. Over a 6 week period of time they can get to the point where they can exercise with a heart rate of 110 to 120 without being short of breath. The total amount of daily exercise does not have to occur at one sitting, and can be broken up into several sessions to make it more manageable.

Why These Operations Lead to Weight Loss

Losing weight is a simple math problem. The number of calories eaten must be less than the number of calories your body burns for fuel each day. These operations reduce your intake of calories through four major mechanisms.

First, all the procedures produce two effects: Restriction and Satiety. The small upper pouch of the stomach, or in the case of the gastric sleeve, the long tube of stomach, will only hold about a cup of food or less at each meal. That means you have to eat small meals, and usually eat around six meals a day rather than three meals a day. You have to chew your food very well, or it takes a long time for the pouch to empty. Doctors now think that some of the nerves and hormones that tell you when you are full are located in the area of the stomach that the upper pouch is made of. This means that just a little bit of food will make you feel full, and many patients have a much smaller appetite after the surgery. By controlling how fast food empties from the small stomach pouch or tube, patients are able to avoid being hungry for longer periods of time. You have very little ability to take in a lot of calories just from eating a large volume of food at one meal, and that meal tends to keep you satisfied for longer periods of time.

Second, malabsorption surgeries, including the malabsorption aspect of the roux en y gastric bypass, reroute the digestive enzymes. This prevents the portion of small bowel that carries food from the small pouch from absorbing the food that empties into it. The bypassed portion of stomach and small bowel has enzymes, but no food to absorb. The lower portion of small intestine that has both food and enzymes will absorb food normally. However, you now have a shorter portion of bowel that has food combined with enzymes, so you absorb fewer of the calories that you eat.

The third reason that patients eat fewer calories is called the "dumping" syndrome. It is a well-known side effect of the roux en Y gastric bypass formation. Eating as little as two grams of sugar can lead to nausea, shakes, chills, sweats, weakness, and a generally ill feeling. It often lasts over an hour, and most patients have to lie down until it passes. There is no way to make the "dumping" syndrome feel better, except to avoid foods that have sugar in them. Most people will not eat foods that make them sick. This side effect teaches patients to avoid foods with refined sugars, which greatly decreases the number of calories they eat per day. Refined sugars are the easiest forms of calories that the body can get. It is important to differentiate refined sugars from complex sugars. Fruits and vegetables have complex sugars, and these do not cause the "dumping" syndrome. The most common source of refined sugars is cane or beet sugar. Artificial sweeteners do not cause the dumping syndrome either.

Since the digestive enzymes do not mix with the food until further down the small bowel, fats are not broken down very well. This is part of the dumping syndrome as well. Bile from the liver is responsible for breaking down any fatty substances in your meal so that those nutrients can be absorbed. But breaking down fats takes time, and the shortened length of the small bowel does not allow very complete breakdown of these fats.

So, if a patient eats foods that are high in fat, the fat is poorly digested. Poorly digested fats can cause nausea, abdominal cramps, and a bad and smelly diarrhea. Most people do not enjoy these side effects, and learn to avoid fried foods like french fries, fried rice, fried chicken, and so forth. The side effects also teach them to avoid meats that are high in fat, like bacon or ham or fatty steaks. Fats are a very concentrated form of calories. On average they contain twice as many calories as sugar. So even though it is harder to absorb the fats, when absorbed they provide a lot of calories in just a small amount of food.

Is just decreasing the intake of calories enough? No. Studies on how people lose weight are very convincing. It is next to impossible for people to lose weight without increasing their output of calories at the same time they are decreasing their intake of calories. Why? The reason is because the body is able to adjust its efficiency in using calories by about 15%. Patients have to eat at least 15% more calories to start gaining weight. They must also eat 15% fewer calories each day to start losing weight. Decreasing food intake is usually a difficult way to lose weight because hunger becomes an issue. After weight loss surgery, patients claim they do not get as hungry. Early filling of the small upper pouch of the stomach stretches the sensors in the stomach that make you feel full. The size of the outlet keeps the pouch full for longer periods of time. For the first few months after surgery many weight loss surgery patients do not experience the hunger common with dieting. If they have an adjustable gastric band placed, it can be inflated further when hunger starts to recur.

So how do you increase your calorie output? You must exercise. But most people go to the gym for a short period of time and torture themselves with severe workouts that they cannot maintain. You do not need to do that. Studies show that you need to burn an extra 200 to 300 calories per day. That means exercising about thirty minutes a day, or walking about four miles per day. Current studies say that you need to do this five times a week. The more exercise you do, the quicker the weight comes off. Even after the surgery you must exercise. If you do not get at least 30 minutes of exercise in at least five times a week, you may lose less than 30% of your excess weight. And if you quit exercising, some of the weight you have lost will come back.

One myth of exercise is that you have to go to the gym and work up a big sweat and a pounding heartbeat. This is just not true. You just have to workout enough to get your heart rate up to 100 to 120 beats per minute. You can count your heart rate at your wrist or in the corner of your neck and jaw. Count how many beats occur in 15 seconds, then multiply by four. This is your heart rate in beats per minute. Try to exercise enough to increase your heart rate without getting short of breath.

It is important to find an activity that you like. It will be easier to maintain your exercise program if you like what you are doing. Some people like to walk, some run, some lift weights. Many patients have pain in their backs or in their knees or ankles. Water exercises are a great way to start exercising and it helps to support your joints. It also provides a graduated resistance to your movements, which puts less shock on your joints. As patients lose weight they can graduate to other exercises. It is also important to try a variety of activities. This can keep you from becoming bored with one type of exercise. Try the treadmill on Monday, do upper extremity weights on Wednesdays, do your water aerobics on Fridays, and walk five miles on Saturday or Sunday.

It is common these days for people to have home exercise equipment. Although any exercise can be used, the treadmill is found to be the most efficient means of exercise. In terms of greatest number of calories burned for the effort, the treadmill is better than a stair stepper or stationary bike.

Walking is a common form of exercise but you have to walk about four miles a day to burn 300 calories. Most patients can not just start walking four miles a day, so I recommend slowly working up to it. I ask patients to walk at least four times a day. Initially, frequency is more important than distance, but to get to four miles you will also need to slowly increase your distance. Start by walking out and back 50 yards each trip. Do this for a week then double the distance to 100 yards. Each week, for six weeks, double your distance. By week six, you will be walking 800 yards out, and then 800 yards back four times a day. That equals four miles of walking a day.

After surgery, patients need to avoid straining their incision for six weeks to allow for strong healing. This helps to prevent hernias from forming. Walking will not strain your incision so it is a good exercise after surgery. Walking also is the major means to preventing blood clots. Clots usually form in the legs when you become less active, and blood clots are the most common reason that patients die after this surgery. Walking will help avoid this major complication.

How Much Weight Can I Lose?

Although there are hundreds of commercial programs for weight loss, the success of these programs is very limited. Less than 5% of people trying to lose weight through any of these commercial programs, vitamin supplements, or medical therapies keep it off. By contrast, surgical treatments for weight loss consistently show success. The least successful surgical treatments lead to about 40% excess weight loss over the long term, and many patients lose 100% of their excess weight.

A key concept in understanding how much weight you will lose is the concept of excess weight. Remember we talked about the Metropolitan Life table for ideal weight. Your excess weight is any weight over the ideal weight for your height. In other words, if your ideal weight is 150 pounds, and you weight 250 pounds, then your excess weight is 100 pounds (250 - 150 = 100).

Patients lose weight according to the percentage of excess weight. It would be unrealistic to expect a 250 pound patient to lose the same amount of weight as a 500 pound patient. You would lose all your weight because the excess weight of a 500 pound patient is more than 250 pounds. Instead, you will lose a similar *percentage* of weight. The 500-pound patient will lose

10% of his/her excess weight in six weeks. At an ideal weight of 150 pounds, his/her excess weight is 350 pounds. 10% of that is 35 pounds. The 250 pound patient will lose 10% of his/her excess weight in six weeks. If the patient's ideal weight is 150 pounds then the excess weight is 100 pounds. They will lose 10 pounds in six weeks. So patients will lose the same percentage of weight but not necessarily the same weight in pounds.

For patients undergoing adjustable gastric banding, it takes about three years to achieve a stable weight loss of 40 to 60% excess weight. For patients undergoing a vertical gastric sleeve, 60% excess weight loss is achieved in an 18 month period of time. For patients undergoing the roux en Y gastric bypass, weight loss in the first two years after surgery is generally in the range of 80% of their excess weight.

After the first two years, some patients will begin to gain some of that weight back, especially if they begin to exercise less. Studies of roux en Y gastric bypass show that in patients followed from 15 to 20 years after their surgery, 80% maintain a weight loss of greater than 50% of their excess weight.

Patients should be aware that surgery is not an instant weight loss program. After adjustable gastric banding, the initial band adjustment does not occur until six weeks after surgery. Only then do patients start to lose weight. And then it takes about three years to achieve a stable weight loss.

After roux en Y gastric bypass, the initial loss of weight is not seen for about six weeks. Typical weight loss is 10 to 15% of a patient's excess weight in the first six weeks. Within three months, a patient may lose up to 25% of their excess weight. By the end of the first year, about 60 to 65% of a patient's excess weight is gone. In the second year, the remaining weight loss is gradual, and most stabilize their weight by the end of two years.

There are patients who fail to lose weight. Failure rates are about 10%. There are several factors that may play into these failures. Psychologic illnesses account for a portion of these failures. Patients can continue to eat foods that make them ill and still get in enough calories to maintain their weight. Patients can eat small amounts of food in a continuous manner throughout the day and get enough calories to maintain their weight. Some patients try to eat large amounts of food, despite having to vomit what does not fit into their small upper stomach pouch. Eventually they can dilate the pouch or its outlet, which then leads to dilation of the small bowel, effectively forming a larger stomach.

It is important for doctors to evaluate the psychological makeup of their patients for any clues that may predict these behaviors or any psychological illness that lead to these behaviors. It is very important for patients to be up front with their doctors about depression, compulsions, psychosis, or addictions that they have had or are currently treated for. Otherwise, operating on such a patient just leads to a life of misery for that patient, and for that doctor. It is not uncommon for insurance companies or surgeons who commonly perform these procedures to refer patients for psychological evaluations and for standardized tests for personality traits.

The Risks of Surgery

It is important that patients are able to understand the risks of surgery and what other possible outcomes can occur. However, it is often difficult for patients to truly understand these risks, what the percentages mean, and how doctors know when things are going right or wrong. It is impossible to list all the possible things that can happen, but the risks generally include bleeding, removal of the spleen, infection in the incision or in the abdomen, hernias, small bowel obstructions, ulcers in the stomach pouches, scarring that narrows the upper stomach pouch outlet, depression, vitamin and micronutrient deficiency, blood clots in the legs or that pass to the lungs, heart problems, and bowel leaks. Adjustable gastric bands have additional complications related to the port that is used to fill the band. It can get infected and have to be replaced, leak and have to be replaced, or flip upside down and have to be revised.

The risks of surgery can be compared to the risks of driving, even if the numbers are not exactly alike. It is not uncommon that you will get into your car and drive down the highway at speeds that can kill you if something goes wrong. Every morning the television and radio programs report on the crashes that do occur, and the deaths that occur as well. We all understand that there are some things that can make driving more dangerous. Driving on bald tires, driving over debris on the road, driving when tired, driving in poor weather. There are a number of things that we can avoid to make driving safe, but even with these efforts, people can crash and can die. People still drive because the benefit of getting where they are going outweighs the risk of crashing. To some extent, surgery is like this. The benefit to be gained from surgery must outweigh the risks associated with surgery.

Your surgeon will interview you to find out what previous health problems you have had, and any clues to undiagnosed problems that can make surgery dangerous for you. Your surgeon may need to do tests or prescribe treatments to help make surgery less dangerous. In the end though, for the patient, the benefit of having a surgery to lose weight, or any surgery, must outweigh the risks. Just like when you drive down the highway to get where you are going, is it benefiting you enough to risk the dangers of the road? No matter how thorough your doctor is, patients must realize that no medical test is 100% accurate, so you will always be at some level of risk for any of these complications.

Risks to Your Life

There are three main causes of death after weight-loss surgery: blood clots, bowel fluid leakage, and heart disease.

Blood Clots

Blood clots can form in the legs, and these are called deep vein thrombosis, or DVTs. They can break off and pass to the heart, then obstruct the lungs, causing death. When this occurs they are called pulmonary embolisms or PEs. They are not always fatal, but when they do cause obstruction of the lung, death is rapid and almost nothing can be done to help.

Blood clots most often start in the deep veins of the legs. Several factors can contribute to an increased risk of blood clots. Smoking thickens the blood and can lead to an increased risk of blood clots. Birth control pills or estrogen replacement medications can lead to an increased risk of blood clots. There are genetic factors that can increase the risk of blood clots, and just being overweight and inactive can increase the risks.

Walking is the body's natural defense against blood clots in the legs. Blood must continue to flow at a minimal rate or it thickens and clots. The feet have a large plexus of veins that pump blood up the leg with each step. The calf muscles of the legs act as pumps with each step to keep the blood moving at a safe rate. Proteins released from the calf muscles with each step act to prevent the chemical reactions that start the blood clotting.

The most important thing that patients can do to prevent blood clots is to get up and walk the day of their surgery. Studies show that the risk of blood clots increases starting after only an hour of inactivity. Within four hours of the end of surgery, patients need to be pacing the halls of the hospital, and walking every four hours around the clock during their hospital stay.

Doctors often treat patients with medicines that prevent blood clots and stockings that squeeze the patient's legs to keep the blood moving. But the risk of blood clots is elevated even weeks after surgery, so a walking program needs to be in place when the patient returns home from the hospital. Walking four separate times a day, about 50 yards each trip, should help decrease the risk of blood clots forming when the patient is at home. Just going to the bathroom or going to the kitchen for water is not far enough and does not count!

Bowel Leaks

Because some of these procedures involve cutting the stomach or small bowel, and then sewing it back together, leaks can occur. The adjustable gastric band is also at risk for leaks if the band erodes into the stomach. If a leak does occur, fluid inside the bowel, which is full of bacteria, can leak into the abdomen and cause a severe infection. These infections can become so severe that they lead to organ failure, including kidney failure, pneumonia and lung failure, liver failure, and heart failure. Any of these can cause death.

Although your surgeon will carefully proceed with surgery, leaks can still occur. Tests can be done to evaluate for leaks. During surgery for a gastric sleeve or gastric bypass, the staple lines and new connections are placed under water, and air is pumped into the bowel to look for air leaks, just like a bicycle inner tube is put into a tub of water to look for leaks. After surgery, patients can be given a contrast agent to drink. If a leak has formed since surgery, it is sometimes seen on x-ray.

If a leak does occur, the patient often has to go back to the operating room for a second operation to fix the leak. It is very important to fix a leak quickly. The sooner it is repaired, the less damage done. Patients can cause leaks themselves.

During the first few weeks, the stomach and bowel are trying to heal the incisions. It takes about six weeks before the incisions are repaired to a nearly normal strength. If patients eat regular, heavy foods, they can strain or tear the incisions if they have not healed enough, or they can tear out the sutures that hold the band in place. Many surgeons will place their patients on a liquid diet that gradually advances to a regular consistency diet over the six-week period to prevent any damage to the pouch or intestines.

Heart Disease

Patients who meet the weight criteria for this surgery (beginning at 75 lbs. over ideal weight) are at a several-fold increase in risk for heart disease. Other factors that increase the risk include smoking, diabetes, high blood pressure, and high blood cholesterol levels. Cholesterol plaques in the arteries of the heart can lead to heart attacks and death after surgery. Your doctor will evaluate what level of risk you have and take precautions to make the surgery as safe as possible for you. However you look at it, the longer you remain overweight, the worse your risk of heart disease. The decrease in the length of your life is directly proportional to the amount of increased weight you carry and the amount of time you spend at that increased weight.

Risks that May Require Further Tests or Procedures

Small Bowel Obstruction

Any time an operation is performed in the abdomen, scar tissue, called adhesions, form. These adhesions can cause blockage of the bowel. It is thought that the adhesions change over time, so the risk of blockage is spread over a person's lifetime. The risk does not change with time, or with the number of operations that occur in the abdomen. The risk after one surgery, like a hysterectomy, is the same after several surgeries. The risk is the same five years after the operation as it is thirty years after the surgery. Usually patients can be treated without surgery, but especially in patients with the roux en Y gastric bypass, surgery is necessary to relieve the blockage.

Stricture of the Upper Pouch Outlet

In gastric bypass surgery, when the limb of small bowel is sewn to the upper stomach pouch, that connection is made to a certain size. In a small number of patients, when this connection heals, the connection can narrow. This is called a stricture and makes it hard for food to move from the upper stomach pouch into the small bowel. It takes too long for the pouch to empty. Similarly, after a gastric sleeve operation, the long staple line can form excess scar tissue, blocking the passage of food through the gastric tube.

In these cases, a procedure called an endoscopy is performed. A lighted, flexible tube with a miniature camera at the end is passed through the mouth, the esophagus, and into the upper stomach. The site of narrowing is identified, and a long narrow balloon is placed across the stricture. The balloon is inflated to stretch the narrowed area to the proper size, and sometimes this requires repeating-several times. In most cases this fixes the problem. Surgery is rarely required.

Wound Infection

Fluid draining from the incision, whether due to infection or not, is the most common complication seen after this surgery. It often occurs after the first week of surgery, but can occur up to several weeks later. Occasionally antibiotics are needed for a short time, but the treatment for this complication is to open the skin incision, sometimes the entire skin incision, to let the fluid drain.

If, after placement of an adjustable gastric band, the port site is infected, the port sometimes has to be removed and then replaced later.

The incision is then packed with moist gauze, once or twice a day, until the body fills in the wound from the inside out. This may take several weeks, and is very inconvenient and time consuming. It is usually not very sore after the first few days, and is fairly easy to take care of once treatment is started. Fortunately, this common complication does not usually cause further problems.

Hernias

In the first six weeks after surgery, your body is repairing the incisions needed to do the surgery. The incision gradually gains most of its strength in the first six weeks, and continues to gain strength for up to a year. During the first six weeks while strength is increasing, your incision is kept closed by suture. Straining the abdominal wall during the first six weeks can lead to tears through the incision. These tears are called hernias. A hernia has to be repaired by another surgery, but it is often postponed for at least a year to allow some weight loss to occur. To avoid the possibility of a hernia, patients must refrain from activities that strain the incision. Lifting more than ten pounds must be avoided. If patients develop a cough, it should be treated with cough medication. Straining to have a bowel movement can cause a hernia also, so constipation must be avoided. If patients develop constipation, it generally means that the patient is not drinking enough water. You can use medications to help relieve the constipation, but drinking more water is a must. Avoid lifting groceries, children, pets, or purses that weigh over ten pounds.

Bleeding and Removal of the Spleen

Because your surgeon cuts through skin, bowel, and other structures, bleeding can occur - generally not enough bleeding to require a transfusion - but your surgeon needs to know if you have any objections to a blood transfusion if you need one. The spleen lies just next to the stomach and is handled during all of these operations. The spleen is a very delicate organ with a consistency like gelatin. It may crack or tear and start to bleed. If it does, then the spleen is removed to prevent excessive blood loss. If the spleen is removed, vaccines are sometimes given to help replace the infection-fighting influence of the spleen. The spleen helps to develop your infection fighting ability during your childhood.

Ulcers

Ulcers can occur after any of the surgeries. Over the counter medicines for pain are particularly common causes of ulcers. Substitute these medications with acetaminophen based medications if at all possible. If not, help protect yourself from ulcers by using acid reduction medications.

Because the stomach is divided into two pouches after gastric bypass, the lower pouch can no longer be investigated. Unfortunately, ulcers can also occur in the lower stomach pouch when patients use these medications. These medications, called non-steroidal anti-inflammatory drugs (NSAIDS) include aspirin, ibuprofen, and other common pain medications. Patients can use acetaminophen, but these other medications are associated with the formation of ulcers, and must be avoided. Ulcers can cause bleeding in the lower stomach pouch, which would be very difficult to find since we can no longer look in the lower stomach pouch, and patients could possibly die from that kind of bleeding. Ulcers rarely form without these medications.

Some would say that a gastric band or gastric sleeve operation should be performed instead of gastric bypass for patients with severe osteoarthritis. These patients often need to remain on nonsteroidal anti-inflammatory drugs to treat their arthritis, and the band or the sleeve still allow evaluation of the lower gastric portion in the event of an ulcer.

Depression

Depression can occur in patients after any major abdominal surgery. For many of our patients, depression is present prior to surgery as well. Ridicule from the public in general leads to feelings of inadequacy and failure. The inability to lose weight despite multiple attempts worsens those feelings. After surgery patients are dealing with a lot of changes. This can worsen depression. Many people turn to food as a comfort for other stressors, but our patients can no longer do this. Their freedom to choose what they want to eat is restricted, especially in the first six weeks when they are on a mostly liquid diet. In the first two weeks after surgery, patients are unable to drive themselves, so they become home bound, and cabin fever can set in.

They are also dealing with the discomfort and restrictions involved in recovering from a major abdominal surgery. So there are a lot of factors leading them into a worsening depression. It is vital that any pre-existing depression is treated before going into surgery. It is just as important that patients understand that the first six weeks are going to be difficult. If their expectations are in line with what their experience will be, then depression is unlikely to occur.

Not eating enough calories each day can cause depression as well. After surgery, many patients lose their hunger and forget to eat. When they do eat, their pouch will only hold a cup of food at a time, so they get very few calories in unless they eat six times a day. It is important for all weight loss patients to eat six times a day to get enough calories in to avoid a depression.

After the first six weeks, patients are over all but minor discomforts of surgery. They resume eating solid food and their regular activities. And best of all, they have begun to lose weight.

Micronutrient and Vitamin Deficiency

All of these surgeries decrease the volume of food you can eat. Many of the vitamins and minerals we need are found in trace amounts in our food. Any of these surgeries can lead to a decreased ability to absorb the minerals, vitamins, and other nutrients that are found in small amounts in the normal diet. Some deficiencies can form because of this decreased ability. The most common deficiencies are iron, calcium, and B-vitamins. Taking a calcium supplement and a multivitamin with iron twice a day usually prevents deficiencies, but it is important to see your doctor regularly to test for any deficiency. Initially you are tested every three months in your recovery period. Later in life you should get a vitamin test at least once a year.

The Risks of Morbid Obesity

Now that you have learned the risks of surgery, you still must consider the risks of remaining morbidly obese before you decide that surgery is too risky. It is much harder to quantify the risks because people that are morbidly obese in their teens face much different consequences than people who are morbidly obese as young adults, and these consequences are much different from people who are morbidly obese in their later years. However, it is overwhelmingly obvious to those in the health-care profession that morbid obesity at any age has devastating consequences. Research has shown that those who undergo weight loss surgery survive longer than those who have the same weight and comorbid conditions but for whatever reason do not have surgery.

Morbid obesity risks include early heart and lung failures, including early heart attacks, congestive heart failure, and asthma as either a new diagnosis or a worsening disease. Hypertension and diabetes are exceedingly common diagnoses in the morbidly obese. Your weight bearing joints wear out early and you develop back pains and swelling in your hands and feet, which can be debilitating. An inability to hold urine when coughing or straining is common. Sleep apnea and the Pickwickian syndrome are among the major causes of death in the morbidly obese. Reflux disease is almost always present. Women suffer from infertility and irregular menstrual periods.

Your mental health may suffer most of all. People with morbid obesity realize that society is unusually cruel to them. They get embarrassed shopping for food or clothes. They avoid social situations, and because of their physical limitations, miss the opportunities to play with their children as they grow.

It is important to understand the risks of surgery so that you make a wise choice about whether surgery is right for you or not. But in terms of the risk of death as well as the ongoing diseases that are associated with it, living with morbid obesity may be a much more dangerous choice. Again, it is hard to quantify those variables to give you a good, balanced number that tells you whether to have surgery or not. The important point is, although it is normal and healthy to worry about surgery, make a rational decision based on the information available, and not an emotional decision based on the fear of the unknown.

Why Are You Having Surgery?

I find that there are four types of patients considering bariatric surgery. The initial group is younger, typically between eighteen and thirty-five. They have not developed serious diseases such as hypertension and diabetes, but are aware that they have been morbidly obese for many years. They suffer from the limitations of the weight itself and find it difficult to climb stairs without shortness of breath. It becomes hard to play with their children because they cannot get up from the floor or get down to the floor to play with them. They may suffer from back and joint pain. Women may have irregular menses and intermittent urinary incontinence. Although they are able to live with these burdens, they realize that as they get older, things are going to get worse. They realize they are at significant risk for developing more serious diseases. These patients opt for surgery because they want to prevent further disease and consider surgery a means of preventive medicine.

The second group of patients may overlap in age, but have had serious disease(s) develop. It may be hypertension in the first few years. More often it is diabetics who want to avoid insulin shots. Although they haven't had their disease long, they have been morbidly obese for years. They have not yet incurred damage from their more serious disease processes, but now look to surgery to help them control these diseases. Hypertension is improved markedly with weight loss, and diabetes is often eliminated. These patients are having surgery to treat serious illness.

The third group of patients have had their serious diseases for a few years and are now having secondary complications. They realize that the diabetes, hypertension, sleep apnea and other conditions are now taking a toll on their bodies. They realize that their life expectancy is now becoming shorter. These patients are now having surgery to salvage what years they have left. Although most of these patients will have a good chance of living at least ten more years, they may not live much longer than that.

The fourth group of patients are having serious difficulties. The disease processes related to their morbid obesity have been present for twenty or thirty years. They have now caused strokes, heart attacks, congestive heart failure, leg ulcers, and other life - threatening illness. They realize that they are now within ten years of the end of their life. These are the patients that are at high risk for surgery. These are the patients who are trying to salvage at least ten years by finally controlling morbid obesity and the complications that occur with it.

Although this does not give you hard numbers to compare the risks of surgery to the benefits of surgery, it does allow you to look into the future to see where you may be next.

Chapter Eight

Getting Ready for Surgery Things to Know

Preoperative Testing

Once you have gone over the information concerning how the surgery is performed, what changes occur in your lifestyle and diet, and what the benefits and risks of surgery are, then you will have to decide whether surgery is the right option for you. If you do decide on surgery, then certain things must happen to get you ready for surgery. What sorts of things are needed?

Getting ready for a surgery usually begins with performing tests in order to be sure that any risks are accounted for. Blood work to look at your electrolyte levels and blood counts are done. A chest x-ray and an EKG are common preoperative tests.

It is common for patients to undergo upper endoscopy to evaluate the stomach for any pre-existing problems such as irritation of the esophagus (esophagitis), irritation of the lining of the stomach (gastritis), polyps in the stomach, infection of the stomach with a bacteria called helicobacter pylori, or damage to the outlet of the chest to the abdomen, called a hiatal hernia. Any of these conditions may change how your surgery is performed or which surgery may be right for you.

An ultrasound is often performed to look at the gallbladder. In order to digest fats, your body produces bile. Bile breaks down fats into molecules that your body can absorb and use. Bile is produced in the liver, and passes to the gallbladder where it is stored and concentrated. Normally the gallbladder squeezes out the concentrated bile when the first part of the small bowel, the duodenum, senses fats in the foods you have eaten. When the gallbladder contracts, concentrated bile is squirted into the duodenum to mix with the food.

When people lose weight rapidly, or gain weight rapidly, it increases the cholesterol and fats in their blood. In turn, it increases the fats and cholesterol in the bile. When the bile is stored in the gallbladder, it is concentrated. Just like salt or water crystals can form as water is evaporated from salt or sugar water, cholesterol or fat crystals can form as the bile is concentrated. These crystals can then grow into gallstones. Studies of patients after this type of surgery have shown that about a third will form gallstones, but only about 3% will need surgery for their gallstones. If they already have gallstones, about 15% need a surgery for their gallstones in the first year after surgery. Your surgeon may place you on a bile salt medication to help prevent gallstone complications. As you lose weight, it will be easier to have a gallbladder operation if it is necessary. In the past, surgeons would always take out the gallbladder at the time of the weight loss surgery, but now that we know the incidence of complications are low, many prefer to wait and see if there are gallbladder problems at all.

Preoperative Nutritional Counseling

Weight-loss surgery in any form markedly changes the way you eat, and what you eat. It is imperative that you get counseling from a dietician or nutritionist to help you understand how to choose the foods you are going to eat. How much can you eat at one time? How do you read the nutrition labels on foods in order to be certain that you are not eating something that will make you sick? What foods are going to help you lose weight? These are all important questions that you need the answers to. A dietician is uniquely qualified to answer these questions, and any good weight-loss surgery program will set you up to go over these issues with a nutritionist or a dietician.

In the first six weeks, you will be on a special diet. There are several variations of the diet, depending on what your doctor and dietician have put together for you. There are special reasons for staying on liquids in the first few weeks. Swelling occurs in the upper stomach pouch when it is operated on, and the staple lines or suture lines need time to heal. The operation inside requires time to heal, just like a cut on your arm or hand requires time to heal. If you stress these areas with solid food, you can cause damage to your surgery. Sutures may be pulled out, a stricture may form, or the pouch may tear. Liquids allow the pouch and small bowel to heal without too much stress or pressure on the connection.

In the first six weeks you learn how much food you can eat at a time. Most stomach pouches are made to hold only about a cup of food per meal. All your life you have eaten much more food at one sitting than this, so it is difficult at first to limit how much you are eating. After surgery, if you eat more than your pouch can hold, the food will come back up your esophagus, and you will throw it up. This can be very difficult if you are eating meats and vegetables. However, if you are taking in liquids when you are on this learning curve, and if the liquids come back up, they are much easier to handle. By the time you get back to eating solid foods, the amount of food you can eat at one sitting should be pretty clear to you.

Your Hospital Stay

It is important for patients to understand how long they will be in the hospital, the events that surround their stay, and the requirements they must meet before they are safely discharged. For weight-loss surgery, patients are usually in their normal state of health, so hospital stays are somewhat more predictable.

For a laparoscopic adjustable gastric band, your surgery is usually a day surgery, meaning you come in, have surgery, and go home on the same day.

For a laparoscopic vertical sleeve gastrectomy, the hospital stay may be two or three days, depending on how the operation is performed, what size tube is created out of the stomach, and any postoperative nausea that may occur.

For a laparoscopic roux en Y gastric bypass, your hospital stay is usually a one night stay, then home the next evening.

For an open operation your stay will last three to five days.

Your first day in the hospital is your day of surgery. You need to arrive at the hospital early enough to get registered, undergo an admission assessment by the nursing staff, and get any laboratory blood work or other studies that may be needed just prior to your surgery. You then go to a preoperative area where the permission slip, or consent form, for surgery is reviewed with you. You need to understand what the consent form says, as this is the agreement between you and your doctor concerning what events may occur during surgery. You should be able to meet your surgeon for any last minute questions or concerns, and you will meet the anesthesiologist.

The anesthesiologist is the doctor who gives you the medicines to keep you asleep during the surgery – a very important doctor!

You will go to sleep before much happens and should wake up after the surgery is finished. Sometimes you will sense the breathing tube that the anesthesiologist puts in so that he can breathe for you while you are asleep. Most people do not remember it, however. You may remember being moved from the operating table to the stretcher that brings you to the recovery room. Once in the recovery room, nurses watch over you in order to be sure that you completely recover from the effects of the medicines given during surgery. They take your pulse, temperature, and blood pressure often. Once awake enough, they start your pain medication regimen. Pain medications can put you back to sleep or even affect your breathing, so initially they have to give you little amounts at a time.

In the recovery room, the nurses ask you to take deep breaths and cough. This is very important for re-expanding your lungs. When you are put to sleep for an operation, the lower portions of your lungs have a tendency to deflate. This does not occur so much when you sleep at home and nap when you are tired or sleep through the night, but the mechanics of breathing are different when you are in surgery. Deep breathing and coughing re-expands these portions of the lung and helps to prevent fevers and pneumonia after surgery. Within an hour or so after coming out of surgery, you will move from the recovery room to your hospital room.

Once in your hospital room, you have an IV running, and for gastric sleeve or gastric bypass patients, often a tube in your bladder. Other tubes may also be present. The drain tube in your bladder lets the doctors and nurses accurately determine how well your kidneys are working after surgery. If you have this tube, it is usually removed the next morning. It is very important that you walk soon after surgery to decrease the risks of blood clots in the legs. Your first walk should occur about four hours after surgery. Then you should walk about every four hours.

If you have had an adjustable gastric band, the doctor will often want to perform a swallow test, called an upper GI study, when you are awake from anesthesia. This assures that the band is correctly oriented, and that fluid flows easily past the band. After tolerating sugar free clear liquids, you can be discharged home. It's important to remember to walk frequently, at least four walking trips a day, at home to prevent blood clots in the four weeks following surgery.

If you have had a gastric sleeve or a gastric bypass, your next day in the hospital is somewhat boring - lots of walking. You will be on IV fluids but nothing to eat or drink until after you have completed an upper GI study. Often times your doctor will let you chew on ice chips, but you have to spit out the water when it melts and be sure not to swallow it. In the morning you will go to the x-ray department to have an upper GI study. This is a test to look for any leaks along the staple line for gastric sleeve patients, and at the connection of the small bowel to the stomach for gastric bypass patients. If it looks normal your doctor starts you on water, then clear liquids. Again, lots of walking will help decrease the risk of blood clots. Although the nursing staff is there to help you, hospitals and doctors often encourage family members to be present and to help you with maintaining a walking schedule. It allows you to spend time with your family while also allowing you to get the medical care you need. It also accustoms your family to your abilities, limitations, and needs once you get out of the hospital. You will need your family's support after surgery, and it is important that they know how to help you.

At the same time that you start liquids, the nursing staff will sometimes also give you medications to help restart your bowels. Normally your intestines have a constant rhythmic pattern of squeezing your food along the GI tract. Without it, gravity could move food and liquids partially into the upper portions of your intestines, but never through the entire length of the bowels. After any surgery in the abdomen, these contractions stop. Sometimes they start right back up again. Sometimes it takes a few days. Rarely does it last more than a week. You have to have these contractions in order to eat and drink, so if they are not working, then you need IV fluids to prevent dehydration from occuring.

Once you start liquids, some medications may help to restart your bowels. Suppositories are often used, and the contrast liquid from your x-ray test will also help. There are three signs that doctors use to tell if your bowels have started to move again. Sometimes your doctor can hear the intestines gurgle when they move. If you pass gas through, then your bowels are functioning. Actually having a bowel movement may or may not mean your bowels are working again, and your doctor will often listen for the gurgles just to be sure. Most hospitals have certain conditions that must be met before a patient is discharged.

You have to be able to get up and walk. It seems simple, but you will need to get up to go to the kitchen or to the bathroom when you get home, and help will not always be there. If there is some sort of emergency at home, you have to be able to get up and get out of the house. You have to be able to at least drink liquids to maintain your fluid levels. If you are unable to drink, you can become dehydrated, which can make you very ill. Most hospitals will not let you go home if your body temperature was above 101.5 degrees Fahrenheit the day before going home. All of your lab work needs to be normal. Although these all seem like simple things, they are important in order to be sure you can be at home alone for a period of time if the situation arises.

If after your upper GI study you are able to walk, tolerate liquids and your bowels seem to be working well, you can be discharged home. Pain is much less and much easier to control after a laparoscopic surgery and patients generally get back their mobility on the first day. Laparoscopic surgery also minimizes the tendency for the bowels to slow down so the contrast x-ray and the clear liquid diet can usually be done one after the other on the second day. This allows the majority of patients to go home on the day after surgery - a major advantage to having laparoscopic surgery.

If you have had a laparoscopic sleeve gastrectomy, you may initially have episodes of nausea. If this occurs, you may just need the anti-nausea medication that the doctor has ordered. If it persists, you may need another upper GI study or an upper endoscopy to be sure that a stricture has not formed. Your doctor will evaluate you for these problems and treat them as necessary, but it often means that your hospital stay is two or three days long.

If you have had an open operation, it may take a few days for the bowels to start moving again. Often it takes three or four days in the hospital before you can be discharged.

After Your Hospital Stay

Once you get home, your recovery lasts several more weeks. You have to remember that some of the risk factors for surgery do not occur until you are recovering. Watch your incision to look for any drainage. It is not unusual for an incision to drain clear or yellowish fluid, or to bleed a little. If the skin near the incision starts to turn red and spreads out like a circle from the incision, notify your surgeon. If you do have drainage, and it becomes thick, sometimes whitish or gray, again, notify your surgeon.

You need to walk frequently at home as well. The risk of blood clots lasts for a few weeks after surgery, and walking helps to prevent blood clots. At least four times a day, get outside and walk up and down the block. If you have a long driveway, then go out to the mailbox. If the weather is bad, go to the shopping center or walk in a mall. A walk should be at least 50 yards long, so going to the bathroom or walking to the kitchen really does not count. If you need to drive or fly a long distance, be sure to get up and walk at least five minutes for every two hours you spend sitting in the car or on the plane.

For the first six weeks after surgery, your body is healing your incisions. It is important to follow the dietary instructions so that you do not injure the stomach or bowel where it was sewn. It is important not to strain your incision, or a hernia may form. Remember, no lifting more than ten pounds for the first six weeks. Try not to bend over or stretch out to reach for things. If you develop a cough, then use cough medicines to help control the cough. Coughing puts a lot of pressure on your incision. So does straining to have a stool, so if you get constipated, you may need a laxative. Most over the counter laxatives are fine, but check with your surgeon. Usually constipation means that you are not drinking enough water. Be sure to get at least 64 ounces of water in a day. Be sure and spread it out over the entire day.

Your surgeon will want to see you back in the office within two or three weeks. Be sure you have an appointment scheduled with the office. After weight-loss surgery, several visits are scheduled throughout the first year to follow your weight loss. You should also keep in close touch with the dietician. He/She can help you to adjust to your new diet. Attend support group meetings to get advice from others who have been through this process.

After weight-loss surgery, there is usually a strict diet to adhere to, especially in the first six weeks. Although there are variations, most are similar to the one described here. You will start off on clear liquids. This means that if you pour the drink into a glass, you can at least see through it to the other side. Water, tea, broths and juices are the most common clear liquids.

By the second week, full liquids can be taken. A full liquid means anything that can be poured into a glass, whether you can see through it or not. This usually lasts through the third week after surgery. Starting with the second week after surgery you will need a protein drink or other protein supplement. Protein is one of the basic building blocks for the body and is necessary for the body to heal and to fight infections. If you are not taking in enough protein, then your body breaks down the protein in your muscles to use. This can make you very weak, so a protein supplement is important. Most patients require 60 to 100 grams of protein per day. This is also a good reason to exercise. Exercise stimulates the muscles to remain conditioned so you do not get tired as easily. Plus, exercise increases the number of calories burned each day, helping you to lose weight.

In the fourth week after surgery, most patients can begin to eat more complex foods. I usually recommend my patients put their food in a blender and puree it so that it still goes down easily. I call this the baby-food stage. I know it sounds bad, but I think it helps patients adjust to the amount of restriction that has been created, and the limited volume of food they can eat at one time.

Your foods will be slightly thicker than a liquid, but still soft enough to swallow without chewing. You can use baby food if you want to, but check the label. Most processed foods, including baby food, have corn syrup added. These become high calorie/low volume foods that can keep you from losing weight. So make sure your baby food has no added sugar or corn syrup listed in the ingredient list.

In week five, soft foods, such as mashed potatoes, are good. Anything you can mush in your mouth without chewing is acceptable. Good examples are cooked peas and cooked carrots and mashed potatoes.

Finally in the sixth week, solid foods can be eaten. It is a long road, and difficult at times with everything else that you have to deal with; but at the end of six weeks, you should already see some weight loss. At the end of six weeks your incision has gained most of its strength, and you can go back to the activities you were doing before surgery. At the end of six weeks you can start a new life.

Other Important Changes

Vitamin deficiencies can be a major side effect of any weight loss surgery. Many vitamins and minerals are present in our foods in only very small amounts. So in order to absorb enough nutrients for our body's requirements, it sometimes requires a large volume of food to get enough of the nutrient into our system. For instance, vitamin K is found in green leafy vegetables. So you have to eat just a certain amount of green vegetables a week to keep healthy. The problem is that with all the weight loss surgeries, food volumes are reduced as a means of controlling calorie intake. So vitamin supplements become a necessity for all the surgeries, or deficiencies will occur.

The most common vitamin deficiencies are in iron, calcium, folate, and B12. If any of these get low, you can develop a low blood count. Studies of calcium and vitamin D show that patients who are candidates for weight loss surgery are often low in both vitamins. After surgery, a similar percent of patients remain deficient in calcium and vitamin D, which can lead to thin bones. So vitamin D and calcium supplementation is important too.

For the rest of your life you need to take a multivitamin, a B-complex supplement, and a calcium supplement. Initially, I recommend chewable, sugar-free vitamins like you might give to your children. An anti-ulcer medication may also be given for the first six weeks. After six weeks you can take any multivitamin you want, and you can quit the anti-ulcer medication unless there is a specific reason you need to be on one.

Many patients take anti-ulcer medications for heartburn symptoms. The laparoscopic adjustable gastric band creates a barrier for acid reflux, and the laparoscopic gastric bypass surgery diverts the stomach acid and bile that cause heartburn away from the esophagus, so you will likely no longer need those medications after surgery. If you do feel fluid coming back up your esophagus, you may have overfilled your gastric band pouch, your vertical gastric sleeve, or the roux en Y pouch and roux limb. Use a baby spoon to eat small bites and count thirty seconds between bites to allow the food to pass through the esophagus to the pouch. After weight loss surgery you have to learn how to eat with small bites, and to slow down when you eat.

You must be careful about the size of medication after this surgery. Pills larger than a plain M & M have to be cut in half or crushed. Capsules do not digest well, and in the case of gastric bypass will pass through without releasing any of the medication, so capsules must be opened and the medication added to your food.

Just like women whose hair thins out when they get pregnant, some patients can lose hair while they are losing weight. The stress of weight loss can cause hair loss. It should grow back as your weight begins to stabilize. Most often patients notice their hair thinning in the third to fourth month, then growing back in the seventh to eighth month. There are other causes of hair loss such as vitamin and protein deficiencies. Your surgeon should monitor nutrients every three months for the first year, then once a year thereafter.

After gastric bypass, the contents of your stomach pouch drain directly into the small bowel, where absorption occurs rapidly.

For this reason, you have to be careful about drinking alcohol. Even after a small sip, the alcohol goes straight to the blood stream and you will get intoxicated very rapidly. If you drink alcohol at all, you must really decrease the amount you drink at one time. Be certain that you had enough water to drink during the day. Alcohol causes you to become dehydrated as well. Since you no longer have a large stomach pouch to drink in lots of water at one time, you have to be careful to get in enough little sips of water.

The small stomach pouch or vertical sleeve after any of the weight loss surgeries will limit the ability to drink carbonated sodas. Even a little bit of soda has a lot of fizz in it, and the fizz can rapidly fill the small pouch. This can make you feel very full and bloated, and can give you gas pains as well. Most people learn to give up the sodas, and it is smart not to try any soda until your surgery has had time to heal. That means waiting at least six weeks, and it is probably better to wait six months before trying any carbonated beverages. In the end, you may want to make up your mind to quit them all together even if it is the day before your surgery.

Even more importantly, the carbonation can stretch out the pouch and its outlet. This means less volume restriction and less satiety after a meal. This is a major cause of weight regain in the years after weight loss surgery. With a bigger pouch, you can eat more. With a larger outlet, the pouch empties quickly and you loose satiety. With a larger outlet you can also push even more food through the pouch and into the small bowel.

Expectations are the most important aspect of feeling happy and satisfied with what you have just done. Sure, you can have buyer's remorse, but this is a short-lived feeling and you want to be satisfied in the long run. You need to know what to expect in order to have the best possible experience with your surgery. Be familiar with the dietary restrictions and then realize that an exercise regimen is a must. You cannot lose a significant amount of weight without exercising. Have a good idea of what your hospital stay is going to be like.

It is important to realize that although the gastric band and gastric bypass surgeries are reversible, the risks of reversing these surgeries can be relatively high. You should think of this surgery as permanent, and the changes necessary in the way you eat are permanent too. It will decrease your tendency to go back to old eating habits.

In the case of gastric bypass, you are choosing to have a surgery that causes you to get sick if you eat foods outside of the diet guidelines. If you eat something that makes you sick, you must learn to avoid that food. If you eat something that you think is within the guidelines, but it still makes you sick, then you still have to avoid that food. It may have been made with sugar or fats that you did not know were used. There is nothing that can make the "dumping" syndrome better. You just have to wait until the feeling of illness goes away.

In the Years After

Typically patients lose weight in three stages. In the first six months, the rate of weight loss is the greatest. During this period of time, the swelling of surgery initially reduces the amount you can eat. This improves in about six weeks, but the pouches are still very tiny, and the sleeve is very narrow. Some stretching of the pouch and the sleeve occurs in the first six months; and by the end of six months you should have a stable sleeve or pouch size.

This limit on food volume helps to increase your weight loss in the first six months. If you have a lot of weight to lose, this is the easiest time to lose it. Your exercise regimen greatly influences your weight loss during this period. Increasing your calorie output, i.e. exercise, increases your rate of weight loss.

In the next six months, the rate of weight loss is elevated, but not as much as in the first six months. You have probably experienced what are called "plateaus" in the first six months. Times when there is little weight loss but usually loss of inches around the waist and other areas. Initially, these plateaus may last a week or two, but in the second six months, they can last three to four weeks. Increasing your exercise regimen and drinking lots of water seems to make these cycles shorter. If you have an adjustable gastric band, and the weight loss does not resume after two weeks, go see about having another adjustment.

Between one and one half years after surgery, your weight loss will slow. If you have had a gastric sleeve or gastric bypass, it is during this time that your weight starts to stabilize. For gastric bypass patients, this is the time that your small intestine is adapting to increase the absorption of the food it sees. Although some increase in absorption occurs with time, you will never absorb food and nutrients at the rate that you did before surgery.

Most gastric sleeve and gastric bypass patients stabilize their weight in one and a half to two years after surgery. Some will even gain five or ten pounds if they start to exercise less. As you can see, exercise is a major theme here, and it really fine-tunes your weight loss capacity.

For adjustable gastric band patients, weight loss continues at a slow pace until the third year. Then it will usually stabilize if your activity level remains the same.

After you seem to stabilize, it is wise to wait a few months in order to be sure that your weight does not begin to change again. If your weight remains stable for several months you may consider plastic surgery to remove loose skin, to tighten your abdominal wall, or whatever other cosmetic changes you feel are necessary. Having these procedures done too soon after surgery, before your weight is stable, risks the final outcome of these surgeries.

Women may consider pregnancy after their weight stabilizes. Often, infertility is caused by the hormonal changes due to morbid obesity. After weight loss, fertility may improve. Pregnancy before your weight stabilizes puts your life at risk, your pregnancy at risk, and may increase the risk of birth defects.

Managing your life after surgery for weight loss is much different than it was before surgery. Consider two years as the time it takes to recover fully from surgery. Take the time to consider the changes in your abilities, your physical health, your mental health, and the way you relate to society and to your family. All these are important when considering weight-loss surgery.

Chapter Nine

Your Eating Lifestyle After Weight Loss Surgery

After weight-loss surgery of any kind, you must make severe changes in the way you eat. Before surgery, you had really bad eating habits. Go ahead, admit it! Now, you have to understand that picking the right foods to eat is a constant decision on your part. However, it is not as hard as it seems. Once you get into the habit of eating the right foods, picking the right foods becomes second nature.

If your operation relies on restriction and satiety only, then you can eat refined sugars and fried or fatty foods if you want. But these are high calorie, low volume foods, and they are going to diminish your efforts at weight loss. So even though you technically don't have to eat the same as a gastric bypass patient, I encourage you to learn and follow the same healthy eating habits, so that you can maximize the success of your weight loss surgery.

For gastric bypass patients, the "dumping" syndrome is a constant reminder, and serves to help you avoid returning to bad habits. Avoid the high calorie low volume foods, or you will pay the price!

Once surgery is complete you will want to follow a diet plan during your recovery process. The recommended diet not only helps you to lose additional weight in the few weeks after surgery, but it helps you to heal as well. There are several types of programs available for bariatric surgery. You can pick and choose from advice in this book as well as from websites and other materials.

Before surgery you will want to eat normally. Eat plenty of nutritious foods to nourish your body. The day prior to your procedure you will want to drink only liquids. This makes it easier for your bowels to return to normal function after surgery. It is a good idea to start taking your vitamins too. Start a month before surgery and take them until the day before surgery. Some of those fat-soluble vitamins remain in your body tissue and can help give you nutrients in the days following surgery. Other vitamins are water-soluble and no matter how much of those you eat, they are eliminated very quickly from your body.

After bariatric surgery, your nutritional needs are very similar to your pre-surgery needs. The only difference is that it is more of a challenge to meet those same needs. The amount of food that you eat after surgery will obviously be limited. Your new smaller stomach pouch will not hold as much nutrient-containing foods. After gastric bypass surgery, the food that you eat is not exposed to as much of your small intestine. The small intestine is usually highly absorptive as far as nutrients go, but the shorter length of intestine can limit how much is absorbed. In other words, your small intestine is shorter and that means that the surface area available to absorb nutrients is limited.

After the surgery you will probably find that your appetite has decreased. Most bariatric patients must remind themselves to eat when they are not hungry. It is very important to eat six times a day after surgery. Because of your small pouch size, you have to eat more often to get a healthy number of calories in each day, and enough of the micronutrients. Some find this to be a new experience, but also a welcome side effect of the surgery. Some bariatric patient's appetites are low simply because of the change in their diets immediately following surgery. You may find yourself eating foods that you never ate before. There is an initial change in the consistency of the food to allow for healing, and this may change the feeling of fullness.

Concentrate on Specific Nutrients

It is important for you to concentrate on specific nutrients after having the surgery. Some nutrients are needed in large amounts, whereas in others, only the tiniest amount is needed to satisfy your body's needs. You need to make sure that you take in enough calories to give your body the energy that it needs to carry you through the day. Protein is important as well as a variety of vitamins and minerals such as calcium and iron. You obtain most of your vitamins from a supplement, at least in the beginning stages after surgery. Later on you are able to get many of your vitamins through the foods that you carefully select.

Protein

We will discuss protein goals first. Protein is important after surgery because it is the basic building block for the tissue that you need to produce to heal. Your muscles are made up of protein and water. When you are lacking in protein your body draws off of its own muscle to get the protein that it needs. In other words, your muscle mass decreases and your fat remains. On the other hand if you eat enough protein your body will use your body fat as energy. After all, that is why you wanted the surgery in the first place.

Proteins have other functions in the body, which include fluid balance, production of hormones, fighting infections, blood clotting, and many others. You also need protein to keep your hair healthy. Your hair is made up of protein stores. Without the needed protein you may lose some hair. Hair loss associated with poor protein intake usually occurs three to four months after surgery. Your hair usually grows back in the seventh to eighth month. Hair loss can also occur after any type of surgery due to added stress on the body. Typically this type of hair loss happens one to two weeks after a surgery and is nothing to be alarmed about.

How much protein is enough? Let's go through that calculation. The average healthy person needs about 0.8 grams of protein per kilogram of body weight. First take your present body weight in pounds and divide that number by 2.2. That answer will be your weight in kilograms. Next take that number and multiply it by 0.8. That answer is the number of grams of protein that you need per day (e.g., a 250 pound person needs 91 grams of protein per day: 250 pounds / 2.2 = 114 kg x 0.8 = 91 grams of protein.)

An important point to remember is that your body weight decreases drastically after surgery. It is necessary to continuously calculate your protein needs as the weight comes off. Dieticians recommend calculating protein needs once per week in the first six weeks after surgery, and then less often as your weight loss slows. Too much protein for long periods of time can be stressful on the body. Recalculating your needs occasionally as you lose weight is all you need to keep your protein requirements in a healthy range.

Protein is probably the most common and challenging nutrient to consume. Your needs are not necessarily higher after surgery, but again it becomes more difficult to obtain the desired amount due to the limited size of the stomach pouch. Unfortunately, protein is not available in a "pill" form like vitamins are. The components of protein are so large that it is not possible to make it in such a compact form. Later on, after you heal, you will mainly get your protein from your diet; but in the first stages after surgery, you may need to find additional ways to get protein in your diet to make up your daily needs. For example, let's say that your protein needs are 91 grams in a day. You might drink a glass of milk, eat a serving of yogurt, and in the later stages eat an ounce or two of tuna. If this were all that you ate during the day, you would find yourself sorely lacking in your 91 grams at the end of the day.

There are several things you can do to achieve your protein goals. Protein powders are available at "Health Food" stores and are probably your best option after surgery. A list of common protein supplements is included in further chapters, and many are available on the internet as well.

Look for a protein powder that has about 25 grams per serving and make sure that the serving size is small. If you find a protein powder that has 15 grams of protein, but the serving size is 18 ounces, it is not very helpful to you because you will have a hard time getting in such a large serving size. Another protein source is powdered milk. However, powdered milk does not offer as much protein as protein powder, but it has an advantage in that it adds good flavor to the foods that you eat in the first few weeks after surgery. The best way to get your protein is to select foods that are high in protein.

Once you are able to eat meats, these will be your most common source of protein. Stick with low-fat beef, chicken, and fish. Most meat has about seven grams of protein per ounce on the average. Dairy products like skim milk, low-fat yogurt, and low-fat cottage cheese are also excellent sources of protein as well. Other foods, like most vegetables, have limited amounts of protein, so they may not be the best source right after your surgery.

Iron

Iron is a mineral that is important for so many reasons. It is needed for strength and contraction of muscles. Your immune system is also strengthened by iron. Iron along with protein makes up a substance called hemoglobin. Hemoglobin carries oxygen to all the tissues in your body. The best source of iron comes from red meats. You can also get iron from foods like beans and dark green leafy vegetables, but your body does not absorb this type of iron as well. Eating an iron-containing food or supplement with a source of vitamin C improves absorption of the iron.

Vitamin B12

Vitamin B12 is found in many of the foods that you may eat. But with the smaller volumes and lower absorption, you may not get enough in your diet. B-12 is necessary for your body to produce healthy red blood cells. Without enough B-12 you can develop anemia, which will make you feel tired and sometimes short of breath. Only about 1% of patients develop a B-12 deficiency after Roux en Y bypass, but since other B vitamins may be at risk, it is a good idea to take a B complex vitamin after surgery. Most patients respond to B vitamins by mouth, but if a severe deficiency develops, your primary care doctor can give you a B-12 shot that increases your body's stores for several months.

Calcium

Calcium intake is important for strong bones and normal muscle function, including normal heart rhythms. Calcium is most often found in dairy products, which are encouraged after your surgery. Vitamin D is necessary for your body to absorb and use the calcium properly, so look for dairy products that are enriched with Vitamin D. Even with Vitamin D, it is difficult to get your daily requirement of calcium from your diet.

One of the major sites of calcium absorption is at the lower portion of the stomach. With the roux en Y gastric bypass, this area of the stomach is excluded from the food pathway, so calcium supplements are necessary in your diet. Most often we recommend Tums® because they are rich in calcium, are easily identified by patients, and are fairly inexpensive. Two Tums® twice a day provides enough calcium. You can use any calcium supplement however, if some other supplement tastes better to you. You need between 1000 and 2000 mg. of calcium intake per day. Avoid taking much more than that because too much calcium in your diet can cause problems as well.

How to eat after weight loss surgery

It is a great shame that some patients undergo weight loss operations without the proper counseling about how to eat after the operation. The weight loss surgeries work only because they cause a change in the rules of the game of eating. If you do not understand the rules, you could spend the rest of your life finding it very difficult to eat.

Rule 1

Learn to eat small amounts to avoid vomiting.

The reduction in your stomach's storage capacity makes it difficult to eat more than a cup or two of food at one sitting. You must learn to eat slowly. This allows time for the pouch or sleeve to empty. You must learn to chew everything to a mush. You no longer have a big stomach to grind food for you. If you fill the pouch with food that has to be ground up, you will be uncomfortable for a long time while the little pouch or the sleeve tries as hard as it can to grind up your food. If you overfill the pouch, the food comes up. It does not go down. A good technique to use is to eat with a baby spoon. Usually, we get up in the morning, run downstairs, pour a big bowl of cereal and grab the big spoon so we can shovel the food down in a hurry. Everyone is in a rush. Now, however, you need to slow down. Use a babyspoon to control the size of your bite of food. Wait thirty seconds between bites to allow the food to reach the stomach pouch. Then you can tell if you are full before you take the next bit.

Rule 2

Eat six times a day to burn fat.

One of the benefits of the small pouch or sleeve is that it fills quickly and you feel full. You will not be very hungry after this operation, and this may last for six months or so. This is not such a great thing. Not eating enough calories is just as harmful as eating too many. I urge my patients to eat six times a day to assure they are getting in enough calories to provide fuel for the body's activities. The calories our bodies burn come in three forms: carbohydrates, fats, and proteins. These are the "fuels" our bodies use to keep us going, and the body will pick which fuel to use based on several factors.

Calories come in three forms:

Carbohydrates (both simple and complex forms)
Proteins
Fats

Just like your car is a gasoline vehicle, and runs mainly on gasoline, we are carbohydrate vehicles and are designed to run primarily on carbohydrates. Your car will also run on ethanol or several grades of octane. Your body can also use other fuel sources as well if needed.

Carbohydrates are sugars, and are present in both simple and complex forms. Carbohydrates that include the simple sugars are store-bought cane or beet sugar, corn syrup that is often added to foods, honey and molasses. These four simple sugars can trigger the dumping syndrome in patients that have had gastric bypass. They are just as important for other weight loss surgery patients to avoid though. These sugars will cause less weight loss because they provide high calories in even small volumes.

Four simple sugars that may cause dumping

Store-bought sugars
Corn syrup
Molasses
Honey

Carbohydrates also include complex sugars that usually do not cause dumping, and are not high calorie – low volume foods. These include artificial sweeteners, sugars found in nature - fruits and vegetables - and starches.

Complex sugars do not cause dumping

Artificial sweeteners
Sugars in fruits and vegetables
Starches

Our bodies prefer to run on carbohydrates when they are available. Our bodies can store carbohydrates in the liver, and this supply can last around eighteen hours. If we do not eat, or don't eat something with carbohydrates, then our body may switch to burning proteins as a fuel.

The majority of our protein is stored in our body as muscle. Protein is used every day for regular maintenance in our bodies. Tissues that wear out are replaced, injuries are repaired, and protein structures help us fight infection. However, if we run out of carbohydrates, then our bodies will break down muscle to use protein as a fuel.

I like to use this example: Pretend you are driving a water truck through the Sahara desert and it breaks down hundreds of miles from anywhere. You have no food but plenty of water so you do not perish of thirst. Your body will first burn the carbohydrates stored in you liver, then start breaking down muscle for a fuel. It is not a very efficient fuel but it works!

Your body will continue to burn protein as a fuel for about two to four weeks. It then will begin to burn fat.

Fat is a very rich source of calorie fuel. Most bariatric patients want to burn their fat as a fuel to lose weight. Unfortunately, that is not what your body wants to do.

Your body will first burn carbohydrates, then proteins, and then fats. It is probably a survival strategy developed over time. Muscle itself burns calories and will burn more calories every day than any other tissue in the body. If you are stuck somewhere without food, it would be wise to get rid of the tissue that burns more calories first. That way the stored fuel lasts longer. Each day you lose muscle, you burn less fuel, and in the situation of being stuck in the Sahara, you will survive longer.

This presents a problem for bariatric patients. If your body uses up muscle in the first few weeks after your surgery, then you get very weak, very tired, and can have a serious depression. Fortunately, science has provided us with an alternative answer. Research has shown that if you are burning more calories than you eat every day, you lose weight either by burning protein or fat. Your body decides on which fuel source by measuring how many carbohydrates you have consumed during the day. If you have about 1000 calories a day in carbohydrate, then your body will prefer to burn fat to make up extra calories needed. If less than 1000 calories, your body will burn muscle first. I guess it is a way for your body to tell if you are in the Sahara–a starvation situation-or if you are just not eating as much.

Keeping the body adequately supplied with carbohydrates is why is it so important to eat six times a day. Most of our food is a complex carbohydrate base. There will be no need to count carbohydrate calories if you just eat six times a day. This way you preserve muscle, which will burn more calories and lead to more weight loss.

You will then turn your body into a fat burning machine.

Rule 3

Avoid the high calorie low volume foods that cause dumping, even if you don't get dumping.

Dumping occurs when your body cannot handle the concentration of sugars or fats in the small bowel. Refined or simple sugars pass too quickly through the bowel into the bloodstream and upset our hormone balance. This leads to nausea, abdominal cramps, chills, sweats, weakness and a general ill feeling. Fats require the enzymes from the first part of the bowel or they irritate the small bowel causing nausea, cramping and diarrhea.

Learn to avoid simple sugars and fatty or fried foods. More than two grams of simple sugars can start a dumping episode. More than 25 grams of fat can start a dumping episode.

These are the high calorie/low volume foods that will sabotage your weight loss efforts. Even though gastric band and gastric sleeve patients do not get dumping, the diet for these patients is the same. Even small amounts of foods that are fried or cooked in oil will have a high calorie content. The goal is to maintain low calorie intake no matter which surgery you have. If you eat foods with refined sugars, these high calorie/low volume foods will keep you from realizing the weight loss you want.

Rule 4

Eat foods that provide protein.

Protein is a very important part of our diet. Protein is the basic building block of the body. Most of our cellular structure is based on protein. Most of our immune function is based on protein. Our healing processes rely on protein. Our bodies constantly turn over muscle and require protein to rebuild muscle and prevent weakening. Since muscle is the tissue that burns most of our calories, the more muscle you have, the more weight you can lose. So you must eat adequate amounts of protein, then exercise to stimulate muscle growth.

Unlike carbohydrates, protein is relatively scarce in our foods. Because your pouch is small, you will have to be aware of foods that are higher in protein and concentrate on eating these first. It is very difficult to do in the first six months after surgery, and a protein supplement is highly recommended.

A protein supplement is highly recommended in the first six months after surgery!!

(yes, I said that twice)

Chapter Ten

Eating in the First Six Weeks

In the first six weeks after surgery, you need to be on a special diet. It is designed to give you the nutrition you need to maintain your health, but to also protect your stomach and bowels while they heal. You will slowly move back to eating foods of normal consistency, but not foods that you have normally eaten before.

Try to schedule eating at least six times a day. This will ensure that you are burning fat to the max.

Avoid drinking thirty minutes before and thirty minutes after a meal so that you can get the right amount of food in. We call this the thirty-minute rule. If you fill your pouch or sleeve with liquid, you cannot eat much solid, which contains the complex carbohydrates and proteins you need. If you drink right after eating solids, you will just spit up what you drink because the pouch or sleeve is already full. It takes time for solids to empty out of the pouch.

Take sips of water from a water bottle every 15 minutes during the day. You need at least 64 ounces of water or other liquid per day to stay healthy and out of the hospital. Avoid using straws, they can fill your pouch with air, and it is hard to tell how much you are drinking at each sip.

To avoid overfilling your restriction, use a baby spoon when you start soft foods and count how many spoonfuls until you feel full. You always want to stop eating before you over-fill. Nobody wants to throw up every time they eat. Using a baby spoon allows you to estimate your meal volume and avoid overfilling.

Use a strainer to strain the solids from soups during your first three weeks. Just drinking water, broth and juice for the first four weeks can drive you crazy!

CLEAR LIQUIDS (WEEK 1)

In the first week, you need to be on a clear liquid diet. Portion size is just as important as what you eat. You will only be able to drink down about a tablespoon at a time. About four tablespoons will make you full. When you start to feel pressure in your esophagus or lower chest, then you filled up into the esophagus, and you need to stop eating until it empties. This may take thirty minutes or more. You also need to learn to anticipate how much you can eat before that sensation starts. Then learn to stop eating before you become too full. You want to avoid having the sensation of your esophagus stretching. All your food choices must be fat-free and sugar-free.

tea, coffee, chicken or beef broth, gelatin, water

100% fruit juices, especially apple and grape-dilute 50/50 with water

Sports drinks (watch sugar content) - Crystal light®, Sugar-Free Old Time Lemonade®.

FULL LIQUID (WEEK 2-3)

You can now advance to full liquids. Full liquids will include anything that you can pour from one cup into another, even if it's not see-through. You will also want to start watching your protein intake. Protein is the basic building block of the body and is necessary for repair of the incisions. It is also necessary to maintain your muscles. Muscles are the furnaces of the body. They burn the calories that lead to weight loss, so it is important to maintain your muscles. Getting enough protein in each day and exercising thirty minutes four times a week are the necessary ingredients to maintaining muscles. You will need to eat 60 to 100 grams of protein each day. Check the labels of the foods you are eating at mealtimes. This is a start towards getting enough protein, but most patients require a protein supplement. You can get protein supplements at any health food store. They come as powders, premixed shakes, protein bars, etc. Watch out for added sugar, but otherwise any of these will do. Have a protein supplement with at least three of your six meals each day.

You also want to start your vitamins. Use a chewable, sugar-free children's vitamin like Flintstones® or Bugs Bunny® chewable. Take two in the morning and two in the evening.

Soups– broth or creamy (strain large chunks at this point)

Thin grain cereals like Cream of Wheat® & Malt-o-Meal®

Baby foods

Skim milk (watch the fat content)

Fat free, sugar free yogurts and puddings

Alba

100% fruit juices, diluted in half with water

Powdered milk (add to other liquids to increase protein content)

Add your powdered protein supplement to foods or make shakes

High Protein sources

Fat Free Carnation® Instant Breakfast

Buttermilk, skim milk, all natural creamy peanut butters

Protein powders: MetRx®, Designer Whey®, Designer Protein®, Pro Mod®, Atkins® shake, Designer Whey®

Sugar-Free Nutritional supplements

Glucerna OS®, Choice DM®, Glytrol®, Resource Diabetic®

BREAKFAST

Cream of wheat

Skim milk with carnation instant breakfast (sugar-free)

SNACK

Protein Supplement

LUNCH

Strained low-fat cream soup

Sugar-free pudding

SNACK

Protein Supplement

DINNER

Strained low-fat cream soup

Sugar-free, low-fat yogurt

SNACK

Protein supplement

NOTE: You may be able to tolerate 1/4 -1/2 cup at each meal, find your tolerance level; stop eating when full!

- Always prepare hot cereals with skim milk for added protein and calcium
- Add non-fat milk powder to foods to increase protein content
- Use a protein supplement that contains ~ 25 grams of whey protein (< 3 grams sugar)

PUREED DIET (WEEK 4)

Pureed foods are basically foods put into a blender. By now you may be able to eat a little more at each sitting, but probably not much more than half a cup. Remember to sip water all day long, take your vitamins, and carefully follow your protein intake. As you are able to eat foods with more consistency, it is easier to get protein in, and you will rely less on the protein shakes. But always be sure that you get enough protein in each day, even if you have to increase the number of shakes you drink each day.

Pureed Foods = blenderized
(everything low fat, sugar free)

cooked cereals	thin grain cereals
Cream of Wheat®	Malt-o-Meal®
baby foods	cottage cheese
mashed potatoes	scrambled eggs
mashed white rice	refried beans

puddings	bananas
lean meats	yogurts
canned fruits	canned vegetables

You can place low fat meats into the blender to puree, or fruits and vegetables. Be careful of the peels, skins, or membranes of fruits and vegetables, as they are hard to digest and can cause bloating, abdominal cramps, and gas.

SOFT DIET (WEEK 5)

Now your list of foods is getting larger, and it may be easier to look for foods to avoid. All of the recommended foods up to now are included. No solid meats, but flaked fish or fish canned in water, such as tuna, is good. No solid vegetables or fruits, continue to puree most of them, but baked squash, baked potatoes, or cooked carrots are good examples.

BREAKFAST

1 soft scrambled egg or ½ cup sugar-free, low-fat yogurt

¼ - ½ banana

SNACK

Protein supplement

LUNCH

2 oz chicken salad (pureed/finely ground)

6 low-fat saltines

OR

½ cup egg salad

½ cup canned peaches (in natural juice)

SNACK

Protein supplement

DINNER

2-3 oz baked salmon or grilled flaked fish

½ cup cooked carrots or 1 small baked potato

SNACK

Protein supplement

NOTE:

- Vegetables must be well cooked and be able to mash with fork into pureed consistency
- Always prepare hot cereals with skim milk for added protein and calcium; also you may add non-fat dry milk powder
- Use a protein supplement that contains 20-25gm of WHEY protein
- Always eat protein food first, and stop eating when you feel full

SOLID FOOD (WEEK 6)

You can now look for food of a regular consistency, but be careful to watch sugar and fat content. You can stop the chewable vitamins if you want and switch to an adult multivitamin twice a day, or you can take one adult multivitamin and one B-complex vitamin twice a day. Avoid beef unless it is already ground, like a lean meat hamburger. Beef is hardest to digest, followed by chicken and pork. Fish is usually well tolerated. Avoid fruit and vegetable skins, peels and membranes or foods in a casing, like sausages–too much fat anyway. Most patients have trouble with breads and pastas until about six months after surgery. They seem to swell and cause pain in the esophagus.

Chew every bite very thoroughly, and only take one bite every few minutes to avoid overfilling. This will allow your pouch or sleeve to pass food. Avoid fluid with meals and continue to follow your protein intake. If you have trouble getting at least 60 grams of protein in per day, continue your protein drink supplement.

High Protein foods

Skim milk

Yogurts

Low fat cheeses

Carnation® Instant Breakfast (low fat)

Cottage cheese

Eggs or egg substitute,

Peanut butter – creamy and low fat

Meats: chicken, tuna, other fish, beef jerky

Beans - be sure they are cooked until very soft

Nuts of any sort, but chew them very well

Any soy products: soymilk, soy cheeses, etc

Beef jerky.

You can always add protein powder to the foods you eat to increase the overall protein content.

You will notice that in the first six months your pouch or sleeve expands to hold a cup to a cup and a half of food, but then it reaches its limit. For gastric bypass patients it is also important to know that the "dumping" syndrome occurs in varying degrees to different people. Some are very sensitive, some are less sensitive, but they all have "dumping" to some degree if they eat foods with fats or simple sugars. You may be able to eat one to four french fries before you become ill. You may be able to eat a bite of cake or even two or three bites; but eventually, you will feel the "dumping" syndrome.

The key is to learn that you do not ever have to eat those foods, and you can not only survive, but also enjoy your meals by making wise choices about the types of foods to eat.

Chapter Eleven

Problems after Surgery

Suggestions for Gas Pains and Bloating

One of the most common complaints after weight loss surgery is excessive gas and gas cramping. Why this occurs is not clear, but there are a few probable causes.

First, many weight loss surgery patients have a lot of reflux complaints. To empty our esophagus of acid, we often "dry swallow", which means swallowing air to cause contraction of the esophagus. This will move acidic fluid out of the esophagus and back into the stomach. All the extra air we swallow causes more burping, gas pains and flatulence. It is a subconscious habit that we learn to break some time after weight loss surgery, when the reflux improves.

Another cause may be a change in the bowel flora. Surgery changes how food is presented to the bowel and sometimes how the bowel is exposed to foods. This may change the acid and base makeup of the intestinal fluid. If this changes, then the amount and type of bacteria may change, even if just for a short period of time. This may cause excess gas production from food digestion, at least until the bacterial population gets adjusted.

Finally, sometimes we are just intolerant of certain foods. Sometimes, this has to do with the enzymes available in our genetic makeup, as in lactose intolerance, sometimes it's the food itself. Everyone I know of has more gas after eating refried beans. So if the food you are eating gives you gas, you may have to change what you eat. Some foods are more famous for creating more gas, such as cabbage, cauliflower and broccoli.

Simethicone helps to prevent gas build up and is found in Gas-X®, Mylicon® and other gas relief products. A liquid form is usually sold for babies and can be added to your water. Put about 5 or 6 drops in a 16 oz bottle of water. Then every time you take a sip you are pre-treating your intestinal tract for gas pains. You can also use laxative suppositories to promote passing gas through the colon. If lactose intolerance is worse after surgery, use Lactaid 100®, Vitamite®, or DairyEase®.

Difficult Foods

After surgery, certain foods may not be tolerated (by causing gas, nausea or blockage of the opening of the stomach). Avoid foods high in fat and foods that are difficult to chew thoroughly in the first six months.

Refined sugars

Eggs

Breads

Rice and pastas

Fried foods

Skins on meats/chicken

Spicy foods

Lettuce

Red meat, beef

Highly seasoned meats

Nuts

High fat meats

Vegetables with tough skins or seeds (tomato, corn, celery) in 1st 6 months

Cabbage, cauliflower, and raw brussels sprouts may cause gas

Food with casings (sausage and hot dogs)

Coarse bran cereal

Coconut

Popcorn

Broccoli

Dried fruit

Orange and grapefruit membranes

Do not swallow gum!!!!

EATING BEHAVIOR TIPS

- To prevent dehydration sip on liquids throughout the day.
- Take small bites of food, chew thoroughly, and eat slowly.
- Chew foods until they resemble baby food before swallowing.
- Do not eat or drink past the first feeling of fullness.

- ☐ Use small utensils (baby plate, fork, spoon) to help with consuming small amounts of food.
- ☐ Drink fluids 30 minutes before or after your meals.
- ☐ Do not lie down within an hour of consuming a meal.
- ☐ Introduce new foods gradually, one at a time, to determine any intolerance.
- ☐ Always eat your protein first.

Grocery Lists for the Recovery Diet

Clear Liquids Grocery List (day 1 thru day 6 post op)

Apple juice 100% (dilute 50:50 with water)

Grape juice 100% (dilute 50:50 with water)

White grape juice 100% (dilute 50:50 with water)

Low-fat broth (various brands, canned or powder form)

Crystal Light® (various flavors)

Sugar-free gelatin (various flavors)

Kool-Aid® - sugar-free (various flavors)

Popsicles - sugar-free (various flavors)

Full Liquids Grocery List (day 7 thru day 21 post op)

(Only use items from clear liquid list as fluid sources between meals.)

Carnation® Instant Breakfast with no sugar added (similar to Alba)

Blended cottage cheese (low-fat, small curd)

Egg substitute (safe if eaten raw in shakes because they are pasteurized)

Hot cocoa mix with no added sugar (add protein powder or dry milk)

Juices only 100% and dilute 50/50 with water

Sugar substitutes

Cooked cereals, baby cereals

Skim milk

Yogurt such as Dannon Lite and Fit® and/or Yoplait Light® (smooth flavors, no sugar added)

Nonfat dry powdered milk (add to everything!)

Protein powder (<3g sugar, ~25g protein, low-fat)

Pudding only sugar-free and/or fat-free

Fudgesicles with no added sugar

Low-fat Soups such as Healthy Choice®, Campbell's Healthy Request® (blend and strain)

Decaffeinated coffee or tea

Crystal Light®

Sugar-free Bugs Bunny COMPLETE® chewable vitamins

Calcium supplement

Milk of Magnesia and Tylenol®

Prune juice (as needed to relieve constipation)

Baby Spoon to help with portion control

Strainer with fine metal mesh or colander

Blender to mix shakes

Pureed Food Grocery List (day 22 thru day 35 post op)

(Anything from your full liquid list)

Cooked cereals, baby cereals

Mashed potatoes

Refried beans (low-fat only)

Baby foods

Mashed cottage cheese (low-fat, small curd)

Egg substitute (scrambled)

Skim milk

Yogurt

Low-fat saltine crackers (chew well!)

Nonfat dry powdered milk (add to everything!)

Protein powder (<3g sugar, 25g protein, low-fat)

Low-fat Soups such as Healthy Choice®, Campbell's Healthy Request® (blend and strain)

Sugar-free Bugs Bunny COMPLETE® chewable vitamins

Calcium supplement

(Anything low in fat and sugar that you blend yourself)

Tuna salad

Chicken salad

Beef stew

Canned fruits and vegetables

Chili with low-fat meat, etc….

Soft Foods Grocery List (day 36 thru day 42 post op)

(Anything from the previous lists)

Canned fruits (in their own natural juices)

Canned vegetables

Toasted breads (thinly sliced)

Pasta (soak well)

Rice

Tuna

Canned chicken

Broiled fish

Regular Foods Grocery List (day 43 post op)

(Anything from the previous lists)

Everything in moderation!

Chapter Twelve

Reading Food Labels

Grab a can of food. It will help to follow the label.

Food labels give you information about the content of the foods you are eating. This is very helpful to you in avoiding high calorie low volume foods that prevent weight loss. These are also the foods that give Roux en Y gastric bypass patients the "dumping" syndrome. After a weight loss surgery patients must make intelligent choices about what they eat. A judgment must be made concerning two questions:

1) Is the food I plan to eat a high calorie low volume and going to cause "dumping"?

2) Is the food I plan to eat going to give me a good source of protein?

To answer those two questions, patients need to look at five separate pieces of information:

1) serving size

2) ingredient list

3) sugar content

4) fat content

5) protein content

You want to evaluate each label you read in the same order and the same way so it becomes a habit that allows you to quickly scan the label for information.

Serving Size

First, what is the serving size listed on the package? All the information about what is in the food is based on serving size. Since most of the surgeries limit the volume of food a patient can eat, sometimes you can eat more than one serving size but usually you cannot. If you cannot eat a whole serving size, then you may have to calculate how much of each ingredient you take in. For instance, if a can of soup is one serving with four grams of sugar, but you can only eat half a can at a time, then you will only be eating two grams of sugar. The difference is that four grams of sugar may cause "dumping," and two grams will not.

Even if you did not have a gastric bypass operation, If you get small amounts of high calorie food in, it's the same as eating large amounts of regular calorie food. This prevents weight loss, or may cause weight gain. So even though we reference "dumping", it means the same to a band or sleeve patient, because the goal is to achieve an eating lifestyle that is the same no matter which surgery you had.

Ingredient List

The second thing you need to know is what are the first five ingredients in the ingredient list. The ingredient list is in order of the most to the least. There is more of the first thing on the list than the second, more of the second than the third, and so on. By the fifth ingredient, the amount in each serving size is small. This is where you learn whether sugars, oils, or fats were added in large amounts to the food you plan to eat. If these are listed in the first five ingredients, chances are this is a high calorie low volume food that prevents weight loss, causes weight regain, and contains enough to cause dumping in gastric bypass patients.

The way sugars are listed on labels can be confusing. Sometimes labels list simple sugars as sugar. Other times they list both simple and complex sugars as sugar. Sometimes they list both as carbohydrates. Most of the time, they list simple sugars as sugar, and complex sugars as carbohydrates.

This is important because simple sugars cause "dumping" and complex sugars usually do not. Simple sugars move into the body very easily and can be quickly converted to fat storage. The ingredient list helps you determine what the rule really is. If the ingredient list has only apple juice listed, and the label says 32 grams of sugar, then you can expect that the sugar is a complex sugar that does not cause "dumping", is not considered a high calorie - low volume food, and will not lead to weight gain. If the ingredient list has sugar listed in the first five ingredients, then the label usually lists both an amount of sugar and an amount of carbohydrate.

There are three basic food ingredients that we are concerned with: 1) sugar 2) fat and 3) protein. The food labels tell you how much of each is in a serving of food. The label also tells you how much food is in a "serving size." You need to determine whether the serving size is more or less the amount of food that your pouch will hold at a single sitting.

Sugars

Simple sugars are what manufacturers add to foods to make you buy and eat more of their product. They also are the main high calorie/low volume ingredients. It is easy to change a nutritious food into a high calorie low volume food just by adding a little sugar. If you had gastric bypass, you are most likely to experience "dumping" from simple sugars, so we will concentrate on those first. There are concentrated sweets, refined sugars, and natural sugars. Concentrated sweets almost always cause "dumping" and include maple syrups, corn syrups, honey, molasses, and such. Refined sugars, like the granulated or brown sugar you buy in the store, usually cause dumping when there is more than 2 grams of sugar per serving size. Natural sugars usually do not cause "dumping" and include Fructose, Galactose, Lactose, Maltose, Sorbital, and Xylitol. Your body gets necessary energy from these natural sugars. Artificial sweeteners generally do not cause dumping either.

Look at your example food label. What kinds of sugars are listed in the ingredients? The ingredients are listed in order of the greatest content. For instance, if corn syrup is listed first, then there is more corn syrup in that food than any other ingredient. How much sugar is in each serving size? If there are more than 2 grams, and the first few ingredients are refined sugars or concentrated sweets, then you should not eat that food.

Type of Sugar __________

Grams of sugar per serving size _________

Fats

Fats are necessary in your diet in order for you to remain healthy; but in excess fats cause "dumping." Fats are considered high calorie - low volume foods, and generally contain twice as many calories as the same volume of carbohydrates or proteins. In general, you want 10 to 15 grams of fat per serving size, or less than 20% of the recommended daily intake of fat per serving size. Greater than 25 grams per serving may cause "dumping" to occur.

Back to the example label.

How many grams of fat are in a serving size? ______

What percent of the recommended daily intake of fat is in each serving? __________%

Protein

You need enough protein every day. Protein is the basic building block of the body. It helps to manufacture tissues that build and maintain muscle. Increasing the muscle mass increases the number of calories you burn every day. Your body turns over protein stores every day as you replace worn or injured tissues. So you have to have enough protein in your diet to support these maintenance needs. If you do not get enough protein in, you become weak, tired, and depressed. If you have not calculated your protein needs yet, now is a good time to do it.

First, convert your weight in pounds to weight in kilograms by dividing your weight by 2.2.

My weight in pounds _________ / 2.2 = _________ kilograms

Then multiply that number by 0.8.

My weight in kilograms ______ X 0.8 = ______ grams of protein per day.

Now look at your food label.

How many grams of protein are in a serving? _________ grams

Some dieticians say that you need to use your actual weight to calculate your protein needs. Others say you should use your ideal weight. If you are a body builder and have a lot of muscle, you turn over more protein and probably need to use your actual weight. If you are a bariatric patient, you probably have a muscle mass more consistent with your ideal weight, so you should use your ideal weight to calculate. Most bariatric patients need 60 to 100 grams of protein per day. Since you are going to eat six meals per day, you probably need an average of 10 to 15 grams of protein per meal. Using a daily worksheet helps you keep track of this information each day. If you are not getting enough protein in each day, you should add a protein supplement. In reality, everyone probably needs a protein supplement for the first three to six months. So go out and try some before it is time for your surgery. Patients differ greatly on their tastes for the different protein supplements!!!

Now, that you have gone over the information on the label, go back and make a judgment. Is the food going to help you or hurt you? Does it provide you with protein or is it just a filler? Is this a high calorie - low volume food that increases the risk of dumping? At first this process will seem tedious, but soon you will start to recognize the foods that you can safely eat and that you like to eat. I tell my patients that they eat in cycles. If you were to write down everything you eat in the next three weeks, you would find that you would have eaten the same things over and over again. The goal of the surgery is to change that cycle of foods. The surgery forces you to make those changes, and learning to read labels lets you make that change intelligently.

Diet Diaries

It is difficult to know if you are achieving your weight loss goals without being able to measure your calorie intake. To do this, you have to keep a diet diary, a record of what you are eating and how many calories, carbs, fats and proteins you eat. Research shows that keeping a diet diary is the most effective non-surgical tool for weight loss because it effects the choices you make when you pick foods. You can keep a diet diary online or on paper.

Use the following daily nutritional summary sheet to help make the changes. I find that patients are better equipped to make the changes if they write down what they eat. It forces you to eat six times a day if you have to write it down; in addition, it forces you to look at the sugar and fat content. It also forces you to be aware of how much protein is in what kinds of foods. Use this for the first six weeks. By then, picking out foods will become second nature.

Daily Nutrition Summary Sheet - Post Op

Meal 1:	Sugar(gms)	Fat(gms)/Daily %	Protein(gms)
________	______	______/____	_______
________	______	______/____	_______
________	______	______/____	_______

Meal 2:	Sugar(gms)	Fat(gms)/Daily %	Protein(gms)
________	______	______/____	_______
________	______	______/____	_______
________	______	______/____	_______

Meal 3:	Sugar(gms)	Fat(gms)/Daily %	Protein(gms)
________	______	______/____	_______
________	______	______/____	_______
________	______	______/____	_______

Meal 4:	Sugar(gms)	Fat(gms)/Daily %	Protein(gms)
________	______	______/____	_______
________	______	______/____	_______
________	______	______/____	_______

Meal 5:	Sugar(gms)	Fat(gms)/Daily %	Protein(gms)
________	______	______/____	_______
________	______	______/____	_______
________	______	______/____	_______

Meal 6:	Sugar(gms)	Fat(gms)/Daily %	Protein(gms)
________	______	______/____	_______
________	______	______/____	_______
________	______	______/____	_______

Daily Totals	_____	_____/____	______

Chapter Thirteen

Meal plans and food lists
By Lisa Badolato, RD, LD

Meal Plans - Breakfasts

	Protein	Calories
Eggs - over easy	6	70
Sausage - round	11	160
	17	**230**
Eggs - over easy	6	70
Bacon - 2 strips	4	60
	10	**130**
2 Egg whites	4	70
½ Apple - peeled	0	37
	4	**107**
2 boiled eggs	12	140
½ Apple - peeled	0	37
		177
Crème of Wheat dry 3T	5	80
Sweet n low choc square	0	130
		210
Special K ½ cup - extra	10	100
½ cup skim milk	4	55
		155
Ins. Breakfast - hot cocoa	10	135
Egg - boiled	8	90
		225

Meal Plans - Breakfasts

	Protein	Calories
Muscle Milk - 1 scoop	16	175
½ banana, s/low, strawberry	0.5	105
	16.5	280
w/ water	16.5	280
w/ milk	4	43
	20.5	323
Muscle Milk - 2 scoops (same ingredients)	36.5	498
EAS boxed shake	15	100
1/2cup oatmeal w/Splenda	5	225
	20	325
Crème of wheat 3T, s/low, choc	5	130
½ cup skin milk	0	80
	5	210

Meal Plans – Snack

	Protein	Calories
Lofat cheese stick	9	60
½ apple peeled &sliced	0	37
	9	97
Cheese whiz 2T	5	90
5 Ritz crackers	1	80
	6	170
½ cup Cottage cheese	13	70
¼ cup 100% pineapple juice	0	35
	13	105
½ cup Cottage cheese	13	70
¼ cup Pears	0	50
	13	120
½ cup Cottage cheese	13	70
½ yogurt	2.5	50
	15.5	120

Meal Plans - Snack

	Protein	Calories
12 Tostitos chips	2	140
Salsa	2	30
	4	170
Cheese: Pepper Jack	9	60
Cow pal Square	5	80
Velveeta Square	3	60
Cheese w/2 crackers	5	110
Beef jerky	12	70
1T Peanut butter w/3 Crackers	7	210
Yogurt	5	100
Yogurt w/crushed nuts	10	300
Power crunch - power bar	7	100

Meal Plans – Lunch

	Protein	Calories
Taco Bell Refried beans	9	90
Taco Bell taco	10	100
	19	190
¼ can Turkey Chili	11	80
4 cracker squares	0.5	32
	11.5	112
S. Beach grilled chicken wrap	12	115
S. Beach southwest chicken wrap	13	125
1 can Chicken noodle soup	9	110
Chicken tortilla soup (Wal-mart)	7	130
Oscar Myer chicken (cut)	22	130
1 can broth	1	20
	23	150
½ can Swanson Chicken	15	100
1 can broth	2	20
	17	120
½ bagel	2	50
1 slice of lite ham	3.3	30
½ piece cheese	2.5	40
	7.8	120
1 Pumpkin Cracker – flatbread	5	100
1T peanut butter	4	80
1/2T Jelly	0	45
	9	225

Meal Plans - Lunch

	Protein	Calories
½ bagel	2	50
w/ 1T peanut butter, 1T jelly	4	125
	6	175
½ can Tune Salad (w/ 1T mayo, 1T relish, 1 egg)	19	140
½ sliced wheat bread (toasted)	3	60
	22	200
w/ bagel	2	50
	21	190
w/ ½ pumpkin bread	2.5	50
	21.5	190
w/ 4 crackers	0.5	32
	19.5	172
w/ 8 Tostitos tortilla chips	1	85
		225

Meal Plans – Vegetables

	Protein	Calories
¼ can Spinach	2	30
½ box cream Spinach	4	90
½ bag Cauliflower	3	75
¼ can Peas	4	60
1/3 cup Peas	2.5	35
½ bag Broccoli Cauliflower Carrots	3	75
¼ can Asparagus Spears	1	15
¼ can Green beans	2	30
¼ can Black Eyes Peas	5	100
1 cup Cheese Broccoli	3	50
½ bag Corn	4	140
Baked Potato w/ fat free sour Cream	21	255

Meal Plans - Dinner

	Protein	Calories
¼ can Salmon patty w/ egg	24	180
3oz baked Catfish	19	120
1/3 package Tilapia (Kroger)	20	100
3oz Oscar Meyer Chicken Strips	21	100
3oz Grilled Chicken	16	100
1/8 cup Alfredo sauce (carb control)	1	55
	17	155
7 large Shrimp (26-30ct) peel/eat	15	100
1/8 cup seafood sauce	1	60
	16	160
¼ pkg Crab imitation	6	90
Gordon's FISH:		
Lemon Pepper	15	100
Blackened	17	100
Garlic Butter	17	100
Cajun	16	100
Southern Fried	5	115

Meal Plans – Treats

	Protein	Calories
Sugar-free Chocolate pudding	2	100
Russell Stover Candy:		
Sugar free Toffee (3)	3	160
Sugar free PB cups	3	160
Chocolate squares	3	160
Skinny Cow:		
Ice Cream Sandwiches	4	140
Vanilla and Carmel Cone	4	150
Carb Smart Almond bar	3	180
Sugar-free Popsicle	0	30
Fudge Sickle	2	35
Nuts	8	190
¼ cup Mountain trail mix	5	150
1 cup Watermelon	1	50
Honeydew melon	1	60
Cantaloupe	1	60
1 cup Strawberries (fresh)	1	50
½ Banana	0	55
¼ cup Pineapple (crushed)	0	35

Protein Sources

Food	Portion	Protein(gms)
Beans, Baked	½ cup	6
Beans, refried	½ cup	8
Beans, black	½ cup	8
Beef, ground	3oz	22
Beef, New York Strip	3oz	25
Beef Jerky	1 large piece	7
Cashews	2oz	8
Cheese (low fat)	1 oz.	8
Chicken (boneless baked)	4 oz.	32
Chicken breast (broiler/fryer)	½ breast	35
Chicken (canned w/ broth)	½ can (2.5 oz)	16
Chicken (deli smoked breast)	2 oz.	11
Chickpeas	½ cup	6
Clams (cooked)	20 small	23
Cod (baked)	3 oz.	20
Cottage Cheese (low fat)	½ cup	14
Egg Substitute	½ cup	12
Egg (hard cooked or poached)	1 large	6
Flounder (cooked)	3 oz.	21
Great Northern Beans	½ cup	8
Halibut (cooked)	3 oz.	23
Herring (Atlantic, cooked)	3 oz.	20
Kidney beans (cooked)	½cup	8
Lentils	½ cup	9
Lima beans(canned)	½ cup	6
Liver (chicken)	3 oz.	23
Lobster (cooked)	½ cup	15
Meat Substitute (Harvest burger)	3 oz.	18

Protein Sources

Food	Portion	Protein(gms)
Milk (skim)	½ cup	4
Milk-buttermilk (low-fat)	½ cup	4
Milk-soy	½ cup	4
Navy beans (cooked)	½ cup	8
Nuts, mixed	2oz	10
Peanut butter (low-fat)	2 Tablespoons	8
Peas - split (cooked)	½ cup	8
Pinto beans (cooked)	½ cup	5
Salmon (baked or grilled)	3 oz.	23
Salmon (canned pink)	3 oz.	18
Scallops	2 large	6
Shrimp (cooked)	4 med.	5
Soybeans (cooked)	½ cup	15
Soybeans (dry roasted)	½ cup	34
Tofu (firm)	½ cup	20
Trout (baked)	3 oz.	23
Tuna	3 oz.	25
Turkey breast	3 oz.	20
Turkey- ground (cooked)	3 oz.	20
Yogurt (unsweetened, low-fat)	4 oz.	5

Protein Sources

	Sugar	Fat	Protein	Calories
Protein Shakes				
8 oz cc skin milk	12	0	8	90
Shake Met RX	1	0.5	21	100
EAS Shake	1	3	15	100
Instant Breakfast				
Hot Cocoa	16	0.5	10	135
Dairy				
Lofat Cheese Stick	0	2.5	9	60
Cheese Whiz 2T	1	6	5	90
½ c Cottage Cheese	3	0	13	70
Yogurt	14	0	5	100
Yogurt W/ Crushed Nuts	14	20	10	300
Carb Smart almond				
ice cream	5	15	2	180
Fudge sickle	6	0.5	2	35
Sugar Free Pudding	2	0	2	100
Egg Boiled	1	5	8	90
Scrambled egg w/ cheese	0	2	12	120
Cracker-Chips w/ proteins				
2 Crackers w/ PB	1	17	7	210
2 Crackers w/ Cheese	1	6	5	120
¼ cup tuna w/ 3 crackers	0	0.5	13	120
5 Tortilla Chips				
w/ Tuna Salad	1	7	2	140

Protein Sources

	Sugar	Fat	Protein	Calories
Protein				
Peanut Butter 2-T	1	17	7	190
Tuna 1/3 Can Dry	0	0.5	13	60
Salmon ¼ can	0	5	12	90
Salmon Packet	0	3	15	90
Low Fat Turkey slices	0	1	4	60
Low Fat Ham slices	0	1	3.3	30
2 Fully Cooked Bacon	0	5	5	70
Beef Jerky	3	1	12	70

Fast Food with Protein - avoid >300 calories per meal

	Calories	Protein	Fat
Taco Bell			
Refried Beans	180	10	7
Crunchy Beef Taco	170	8	10
Taco Salad w/o Shell	490	24	25
Tostada	260	11	10
Long John Silvers			
Baked Cod Filet	120	22	5
Fried Cod Filet	260	12	16
Chicken Plank	140	8	8
3 Pieces of Shrimp	135	8	8
Clam Chowder	220	9	10
Lobster Stuffed Crab Cake	170	6	9
Wendy's			
Chili- Small	220	6	6
Baked Potato			
Sour Cream/Butter	320	4	4
Baked Potato - Plain	270	0	3
- Cheese	340	8	6
½ Grilled Chicken Sandwich	185	16	4
½ Crispy Chicken Sandwich	190	10	14
Side Salad	35	1	0
Caesar Salad	80	6	4

	Calories	Protein	Fat
Whataburger			
½ Breakfast on a bun – Bacon	200	8	11
½ Grilled Chicken Sandwich	230	16	9
Grilled Chkn Salad	230	23	7
WAB Hamburger Patty no bun x vegs	300	27	16
2 Chicken Strips	390	18	25
Chilis			
3-4 Hot Wings w/ Celery	550	27	11
Kids grilled chicken- vegs	150	26	3
Kids BBQ ribs w/ fries	370	26	9
½ Chicken Fajita Platter- no tortillas	165	20	6
½ Shrimp & Chicken meal w/ veg	380	31	5
On The Border			
Tortilla Soup	350	14	9
½ Fajita w/ corn tortilla	386	23	9

High Protein Shake Recipes

Berry Berry

½ cup skim milk

5 strawberries, fresh or frozen, no added sugar

¼ cup frozen raspberries, no added sugar

½ cup yogurt, no added sugar

1 scoop protein powder (unflavored or vanilla)

Key Lime Pie

6 oz key lime pie yogurt, no sugar added
1/8 cup skim milk
1 tbsp sugar free lime jello
1 scoop protein powder (unflavored)
½ graham cracker

Chocolate Banana

1/3 cup skim milk
2 tbsp sugar free chocolate syrup
½ banana
1 scoop chocolate protein powder
3-4 ice cubes

Fruit Ice

½ cup skim milk
5 frozen strawberries, no added sugar
2 frozen peaches, no added sugar
¼ cup crushed pineapple, packed in natural juice
1 scoop protein powder

Pineapple Smoothie

6 oz skim milk
¼ cup crushed pineapple
1 scoop protein powder (banana creme or vanilla flavor)

Blend in blender on high for ~ 1 minute.

Vitamin and Mineral Supplementation

Although vitamins and mineral do not provide energy, they are essential for the body to function properly and utilize the energy found in foods. After surgery it is essential that you supplement your diet with vitamins and minerals. It is very important that you take your supplements every day and for the rest of your life!

Vitamin and mineral supplementation recommendations and doses may vary between bariatric centers so be sure to follow your surgeon or dietitians recommendations. Specialized bariatric products are available.

Suggested Postoperative Vitamin Supplementation

Roux en Y Gastric Bypass

2 Adult Multivitamins with iron per day

(200% of daily value)

- Begin with chewable or liquid, advance to whole tablet as directed by surgeon

Vitamin B12

- 1000 µg/month- Intramuscular injection
- 350-500µg/day-Oral (sublingual, liquid drops, mouth spray, nasal gel/spray)

Calcium

- Calcium 1500-2000 mg/day
- Available in various forms. Calcium Citrate or Calcium Carbonate (Tums®)

    - Although studies are limited Calcium Citrate with Vitamin D3 may be the preferred form for the most effective absorption
- Begin with chewable or liquid, advance as directed by surgeon
- Do not take with iron supplement
- Split into 500-600 mg doses

Iron

- Minimum of 18-27mg/day elemental
- Recommended for menstruating women
- Begin with chewable or liquid, advance as directed by surgeon
- Do not take with calcium supplements (take > 2 hours apart)
- Vitamin C may enhance absorption

B complex (optional)

- B50 – 1 daily

Laparoscopic adjustable gastric band (Lap Band)

1 Adult Multivitamin with iron daily

(100% of daily value)

- Begin with chewable or liquid, advance to whole as directed by surgeon

Calcium

- Calcium 1500-2000 mg/day
- Available in various forms. Calcium Citrate or Calcium Carbonate (Tums®)

  Although studies are limited Calcium Citrate with Vitamin D3 may be the preferred form for the most effective absorption
- Begin with chewable or liquid, advance as directed by surgeon
- Do not take with iron supplement
- Split into 500-600 mg doses

B complex (optional)

- B50 –1 daily

Sample Vitamin Schedule for postoperative Roux en Y gastric bypass patient

Breakfast: Multivitamin and Calcium supplement

Lunch: B12 and Calcium supplement

Dinner: Multivitamin and Calcium supplement

Bedtime: Iron supplement (if prescribed)

References: L. Aills et al. / Surgery for Obesity and Related Diseases 4 (2008) S73-S108.

Chapter Fourteen

Protein Supplements

Isopure (2 Scoops)

Flavors: Chocolate, Vanilla, & Strawberry

200 Calories	0gm Fat
0gm Sugar	50 Gm Protein
0gm Fiber	Vitamins & Minerals

New Whey – 1 Vial (3.1 Fluid Ounces)

Flavors: Blue Raspberry, Grape, Orange, & Fruit Punch

176 Calories	0gm Fat
0gm Fiber	42 gm Protein
2gm Carbs	0gm Sugar

Muscle Milk (1 Shake)

Flavors: Banana Crème, Vanilla Crème, & Chocolate Milk

350 Calories	2gm Fiber
7gm Sugar	34gm Protein
17gm Fat	Vitamins & Minerals

Designer Whey (www.designerwhey.com)

Flavors: Chocolate, chocolate Peanut Carmel, Strawberry, French Vanilla, Tropical Punch, Natural, & Vanilla Praline

90 Calories	0gm Fiber
1.5gm Fat	18gm Protein
2gm Sugar	Vitamins & Minerals

Met-Rx Original Drink Mix

Flavors: Original, Vanilla, & Extreme Chocolate

260 Calories	18gm Total Carbs
40gm Protein	2gm Fiber
3gm Sugar	

Promod Protein Powder (1Scoop)

28 Calories	0.6gm Fat
5gm Protein	0.67gm Carbs

Choice DM

Flavors: Chocolate & Vanilla

220 Calories	3gm Fiber
9gm Protein	11gm fat
24gm Carbs	Vitamins & Minerals

Resources Diabetic (7.9 Fluid Ounces)

Flavors: French Vanilla, Classic Chocolate, Creamy Strawberry

250 Calories	3gm Fiber
15gm Protein	11gm Fat
23gm Carbs	Vitamins & Minerals

Glytrol (8.3 Fluid Ounces)

250 Calories	12gm fat
11gm Protein	Vitamins & Minerals
25gm Carbs	

Cytoplex (1 Package)

41gm Protein	21Carbs
2gm Fat	Vitamins & Minerals

EAS – Myoplex Products

Myoplex Deluxe Bars (1bar-90g)

Flavors: Chocolate Chip, Chocolate Peanut Butter, Cookies N Cream, & S'Mores

340 Calories	7gm Fat
24gm Protein	Vitamins & Minerals

Myoplex Carb Sense Bars (1bar-70g)

Flavors: Chocolate Chip Brownie, Cookies N Cream, Chocolate Peanut Butter, & Chocolate Dipped Strawberry

250 Calories	6gm Fat
1gm Sugar	30gm Protein
2gm Fiber	Vitamins & Minerals

Myoplex Lite Bars (1bar-56g)

Flavors: Caramel Apple Crisp, Chocolate Chip, Cinnamon Roll Crisp, Peanut Butter Crisp, Peanut Caramel Crisp, & Toffee Crunch

190 Calories	4gm Fat
27gm Carbs	1g Fiber
18gm Sugar	15gm Protein

Myoplex Power (76g)

Flavors: Chocolate, Vanilla, Strawberry, Chocolate Peanut Butter, Chocolate Mocha, Chocolate Mint, Rich Dark Chocolate, Banana Cream Pie, Pina Colada, & Peaches N Cream

280 Calories	3gm Fat
23gm Carbs	3gm Fiber
2gm Sugar	42gm Protein

Myoplex Carb Control Ready to Drink (11oz Can)

Flavors: Chocolate, & Strawberry

150 Calories	3.5 Fat
0.5gm Fiber	<1gm Sugar
25gm Protein	Vitamins & Minerals

Myoplex Lite Ready to Drink (11ozCan)

Flavors: Chocolate Fudge, Strawberry, & Vanilla

190 Calories	2.5gm Fat
20gm Fiber	1gm Sugar
25gm Protein	Vitamins & Minerals

GLUCERNA® SHAKES

Complete, Balanced Nutrition® for People with Diabetes

If you have diabetes, maintaining a healthy balance of blood glucose (sugar) levels can make your day-to-day living so much easier. Glucerna Shake is a healthy blend of complex carbohydrates, dietary fiber, and fructose, the simple carbohydrate that makes fruit sweet. Working together, the carbohydrates in Glucerna Shake release glucose into the bloodstream at a slower rate than standard liquid nutritional supplements.

Flavors: Vanilla, Chocolate, Strawberry, Butter Pecan

Lactose-free. Gluten-free. Kosher.

Appropriate for low-cholesterol diets.

Usage:

Glucerna Shake is a great-tasting beverage specifically designed for people with diabetes. It has clinically demonstrated a lower blood glucose response when compared to a standard nutritional beverage.[1] Use under medical supervision.

- For people with diabetes or abnormal glucose tolerance
- For anyone who would benefit from a low-carbohydrate, modified -fat formula.

GLUCERNA® SHAKES

Features:

- Complete, balanced nutrition
- For use as a snack, supplement, or meal replacement in conjunction with the prescribed diet
- For oral use only-not for tube feeding
- Provides at least 25% of the DV for 24 essential vitamins and minerals in one 8 fl oz serving
- Fortified beyond 25% of the DV for the antioxidant vitamins C and E, and for vitamins B6, B12, folate, and chromium
- Meets American Heart Association (AHA) recommendations[2] for fatty acid profile; high in monounsaturated fatty acids
- Contains a unique blend of slow-digesting carbohydrates that has clinically shown a lower blood glucose response compared to a standard nutritional beverage[1]
- Contains 3 g dietary fiber per 8 fl oz serving
- Lactose- and gluten-free
- **Nutrient Profile per 8 fl oz: Calories 220, Protein (% Cal) 18, Total Fat (% Cal) 35, Carbohydrate (% Cal) 47**

Diabetic Exchanges

1 starch

1 low-fat milk

½ fat

Atkins™ Ready-To-Drink Shakes

Description:

Super-convenient, super-delicious, and super-good for you! High in protein to keep your energy up; with calcium, 18 essential nutrients, and absolutely no sugar added! New Atkins™ Ready-To-Drink Shakes will satisfy your appetite on-the-go, around the clock. Keep several cans in your desk at work, more in your locker at the gym, and stock up your fridge to enjoy a frosty, frothy taste treat whenever you need a pick-me-up…or a replacement meal.

Nutrition Facts:

Serving Size (can) 1

Servings Per 1

Calories 170

Fat Calories 80

Total Fat (g) 9

Sat. Fat (g) 2

Cholesterol (mg) 15

Sodium (mg) 140

Potassium (mg) 550

Total Carbs (g) 5

Dietary Fiber (g) 3

Sugars (g) 2

Proteins (g) 20

Atkins™ Ready-To-Drink Shakes

Ingredient Details:

Water, calcium caseinate, soybean oil, whey protein concentrate, cocoa (processed with alkali), cellulose gel, contains 0.5% or less of the following: potassium phosphate, cellulose gum, soy lecithin, natural and artificial flavor, carrageenan, sucralose (a non-nutritive sweetener), magnesium chloride, magnesium phosphate, tricalcium phosphate, d-biotin, d-calcium pantothenate, folic acid, niacinamide, pyridoxine hydrochloride, sodium ascorbate, thiamin mononitrate, vitamin A palmitate, vitamin B12, riboflavin, vitaminE acetate, vitamin K1, chromium chloride, copper sulfate, ferrous sulfate, manganese sulfate, potassium chloride, potassium citrate, sodium iodide, sodium citrate, sodium molybdate, sodium selenite, zinc sulfate, maltodextrim.

Flavors: Chocolate Royale, Chocolate, Vanilla, Strawberry, Café AuLait

Orange Flavor Fruit Drink Liquid Concentrate by Bariatrix

Serving Size	1 Packet .7 Oz.
Servings Per Container	7 Packets per box
Amount Per Serving:	
Total Calories	70 Calories
Calories From Fat	10 Calories
Total Fat	1 g
Saturated Fat	0.5 g
Cholesterol	10 mg
Sodium	40 mg
Potassium	60 mg
Total Carbohydrates	2 g
Dietary Fiber	0 g
Sugars	0 g
Protein	15 g

Ingredients:

Hydrolyzed Gelatin, Whey Protein Concentrate, Citric Acid, Natural Flavors, Contains 2 Percent Or Less Of Orange Juice Solids, Turmeric Oleoresin Color, Potassium Citrate, Aspartame, Canthaxanthin Color, Lecithin

Flavors: Grapefruit, Peach Mango, Lemon, Grape, Pineapple Orange, Wildberry Passion

Chocolate Protimax Pudding or Shake Drink Mix

Serving Size	1 Packet
Servings Per Container	7
Amount Per Serving:	
Calories	100
Calories From Fat	20
Total Fat	2g
Saturated Fat	0.5g
Cholesterol	Less than 5 mg
Sodium	260mg
Potassium	180mg
Total Carbohydrates	6g
Dietary Fiber	1g
Sugars	2g
Protein	15g
Iron	25% (Based on a 2,000 Calorie Diet)
Vitamin A	20% (Based on a 2,000 Calorie Diet)
Calcium	25% (Based on a 2,000 Calorie Diet)
Vitamin C	30% (Based on a 2,000 Calorie Diet)

Chocolate Protimax Pudding or Shake Drink Mix

Ingredients: Calcium Caseinate, Vegetable Oil Preparation (Sunflower Oil, Maltodextrin, Sodium Caseinate, Mono and Di-Glycerides, Lecithin, Mixed Tocopherols, Silicon Dioxide), Alkalized Cocoa, Fructose, Maltodextrin, Salt. Contains 2 percent or less of: Cellulose Gel, Cellulose Gum, Dipotassium Phosphate, Aspartame (non nutritive sweetener), Magnesium Phosphate, Magnesium Oxide, Natural and Artificial Flavors, Silicon Dioxide, Vitamin C, Vitamin E, Vitamin A Palmitate, Niacinamide, Zinc Sulfate, Reduced Iron, Copper Gluconate, D Calcium Pantothenate, Vitamin D#, Pyridoxine Hydrochloride, Riboflavin, Thiamine Mononitrate, Vitamin B12, Folic Acid, Biotin, Potassium Iodide.

Check website for other flavors.

Myoplex Original 20pk by EAS

It takes a solid nutritional foundation to build your best body ever. Myoplex is designed to take the guesswork out of high performance nutrition, delivering the highest quality protein, carbohydrates, vitamins and minerals. Perfect for adding or replacing 2-3 meals a day, Myoplex supplies:

* 42g protein complex to support lean mass

* Good source of 28 vitamins and minerals

* Convenient, great-tasting performance nutrition

Serving Size: 1 packet (76 g)

Each serving provides: Calories 280 Total Fat 2 g Sugars 3 g Saturated Fat 1 g Cholesterol 15 mg Total Carbohydrates 24 g Sodium 330 mg Potassium 550 mg Dietary Fiber <1 g Protein 42 g

Nutrition facts vary slightly with each flavor.

Myoplex Original 20pk by EAS

Ingredients: MyoPro. (unique blend of whey-protein concentrate from specially filtered and ion-exchanged whey protein, calcium caseinate, milk-protein isolate, taurine, L-glutamine, sodium caseinate, egg albumin, and calcium alpha-ketoglutarate [AKG]), maltodextrin, corn syrup solids, vitamin and mineral blend (potassium chloride, disodium phosphate, calcium phosphate, magnesium oxide, potassium citrate, potassium phosphate, choline bitartrate, beta-carotene, ascorbic acid, dl-alpha-tocopheryl acetate, ferrous fumarate, molybdenum amino acid chelate, boron proteinate, manganese gluconate, selenium amino acid chelate, niacinamide, zinc oxide, d-calcium pantothenate, chromium citrate, copper sulfate, Vitamin A palmitate, pyridoxine hydrochloride, riboflavin, thiamin hydrochloride, Vitamin D3, folic acid, biotin, potassium iodide, and cyanocobalamin), natural and artificial flavors, cellulose gum, salt, sunflower oil, salt, mono and diglycerides, sucralose, medium chain triglycerides and soy lecithin.

Ingredients vary slightly with each flavor.

Flavors: vanilla cream, chocolate cream, strawberry cream, tropical variety, orange jubilee, chocolate peanut butter

Recommended use: For a rich, creamy shake, combine contents of each packet with 15 oz of cold water or skim milk and thoroughly mix in a blender or shaker for 45 seconds. Use 2 to 3 servings daily.

Shopping List

Protein supplement: Whey or Soy based

Name: ____________Serving size: _______

Protein grams per serving: _______

Baby spoons Strainer for soup

Mylicon for gas pains

Ducolax suppositories for gas pains

Listerine Breath Strips

3 cases of bottled water - 16 oz bottles

Children's chewable multivitamins - sugar-free

Zantac 150 (generic is ranitidine)

one tablet twice a day for six weeks = 84 tablets

Liquid Tylenol® (acetominophen)

Liquid cold & sinus medicine with acetominophen

Chicken and beef broths, 100% fruit juices, sugar-free

Popsicles Crystal Light

Skim Milk Diet V8 Splash

Carnation Instant Breakfast - Sugar Free

Sugar Free Jello and Sugar Free Pudding

Blended sugar free/fat free yogurt

Exercise regimens Before and after Weight Loss Surgery

Introduction

When you decide to have weight loss surgery, you want to get the most out of your efforts. Surgery will provide the tools you need to make changes in the way you eat, which will markedly reduce the calories you take in. The other side of the equation is increasing the number of calories you burn every day. To do this you need two things.

First, increase your total lean body mass - grow your muscles. The more muscle you have, the more calories you burn every day. You need extra protein in your diet, usually in the form of protein supplements or protein rich foods, to provide the raw material for building more muscle mass. Exercise will then stimulate the growth of more muscle mass, which will burn more calories around the clock.

Second, exercise regularly to maintain the muscle and to burn extra calories. You need an exercise program above and beyond your day to day activities.

To accomplish this, we need to ramp up from a minimal amount of exercise to exercising at least 30 minutes a day. We want to perform aerobic exercise, which means increasing your heart rate to about 110 to 120 beats per minute, but not getting short of breath.

Before surgery

If you don't exercise regularly then try this as a ramp up program. It involves walking four times a day. Break up your exercise into these four walking trips so that you don't try to do too much at once.

Find a nearby track or just measure the distance in your yard or drive

Week One: Walk fifty (50) yards out then back. Do this four times a day each day.

Week Two: Walk 100 yards out and back four times a day

Week Three: Walk 200 yards out and back four times a day

Week Four: Walk 400 yards out and back four times a day

Week Five: Walk 800 yards out and back four times a day

Week Six: You are now walking enough to burn 300 calories a day, the recommended calorie output to maximize your weight loss.

If you are able to use a nearby school track then you have premeasured distances.

Week One: Walk one of the straightaways four times a day

Week Two: Walk halfway around the track four times a day

Week Three: Walk a complete circle around the track four times a day

Week Four: Walk two laps around the track twice. Do this four times a day

Week Five: Walk four laps around the track four times a day.

Week six: You are now walking enough to burn 300 calories a day, the recommended calorie output to maximize you weight loss.

After surgery

A leading risk of surgery is the risk of blood clots. This risk will last for a few weeks after surgery, well after you have left the hospital. Walking is how we prevent blood clots, so we want to use walking as an exercise program in the first six weeks after surgery.

Use the above described walking program for the first six week after surgery.

After the first six weeks, you may want a more efficient exercise program. It ends up taking a lot of time to do all that walking for the long term. A more efficient exercise program is an aerobic exercise program. One that increases your heart rate to 110 to 120 beats per minute, but doesn't make you short of breath. It takes about 30 minutes of aerobic exercise to burn 300 calories. It can be a treadmill, a bike, a weight lifting program, water aerobics, jazzercise or any other activity you like to do. It is important to do something you like to do or you will end up quitting.

Something easy to do is a light upper extremity weight lifting program. We could all use more strength in our upper extremities anyway. You can do this every morning when you get up, or every evening before you go to bed. Get a 3 lb, a 5 lb, and a 10 lb dumbbell. There are four upper extremity exercises to try.

The first exercise is an arm curl. The second exercise is a straight arm lift, from straight down to straight out to the side. The third exercise is a straight arm lift, from straight down to straight out forward. The fourth exercise is a military press.

Hold your weights at the shoulder then straighten your arms above your head.

Do 10 repetitions of each exercise. Use the heavier weight for the curls and presses. Use the lightest weights for the straight arm lifts. Be careful not to use weights that are too heavy for your current strength. Repeat the four exercises four times. By the end of the program you will have spent about 30 minutes, and will have had the right amount of exertion.

Chapter Fifteen

Consultation Forms

Included below are the forms that help you work through the complex process of being evaluated and preparing for weight-loss surgery. They include a weight loss history worksheet (This is something you will have to fill out accurately if you want your insurance company to consider covering your surgery). These forms also include a workup checklist, a reminder sheet of things to get done before a weight-loss surgery, a consultation pretest to check your knowledge of the surgery you are going through, and a standard set of discharge instructions to answer common questions that come up after you go home from surgery.

Weight Loss Expectations

Expectation	Description
Dream weight ____________	"A weight you would choose if you could weigh whatever you wanted."
Happy weight ____________	"This weight is not as ideal as the first one. It is a weight, however, that you would be happy to achieve."
Acceptable weight ____________	"A weight that you would not be particularly happy with, but one that you could accept, since it is less than your current weight."
Disappointed weight ____________	"A weight that is less than your current weight, but one that you could not view as successful in any way. You would be disappointed if this were your final weight after the program."

How do you expect surgery to help you?

Please rank these statements: 1 being the most important and 8 being the least

_____ Improved overall medical condition

_____ Improved overall quality of life

_____ Less pain

_____ Increased mobility

_____ Improved self esteem

_____ Improved relationships

_____ Improved work life

_____ All the above

Previous Weight Loss Programs

(Circle answers.)

Jenny Craig	Weight Watchers
Doctors Clinic	Nutrisystem
LA weight loss	Optifast
TOPS	Pritikin
Atkins	Cabbage Diet
Grapefruit diet	Metabolife
Herbalife	Slim Fast
Medifast	Liquid diet

Others: ______________________________

Medications taken for weight loss? (Circle answers.)

Amphetamines
Phentermine (Adipex, Fastin, Pondimen)Phen-Fen
Redux (Dexfenfluramine)
Xenical (Orlistat)
Meridia (Sibutramine)
Others: ______________________________

Non-dietary therapies: (Circle answers.)

Exercise/Health Club Membership

Hypnosis

Behavior Modifications

Acupuncture

Previous Weight Loss Programs

1. How many years have you been at least 100 lbs overweight? ___________

2. Primary Care Physician (PCP): ______________

3. Date of first exam: ________________________

4. Have you discussed your weight with your PCP? Y / N

5. How much weight have you lost since first seeing your PCP? ______________________________

6. How much weight have you gained or regained since first seeing your PCP? ________________

7. Any other physicians you have seen regarding you weight? ________________________________

8. How many years overall have you been trying to lose weight? ____________________________

9. In that time, how much total weight have you lost? ______________________________________

10. How much have you regained? _____________

Consultation Information Pretest

Name: ______________________________ **Date:** ________

1. Write a brief summary of why you want to undergo the risk of surgery to lose weight?

____

____

____

____

____

____

____

____

2. What is your "Ideal Weight" ________

3. What is your "Excess Weight" ________

4. How much of your "Excess Weight" do you expect to lose? ______%

5. What are the three main risks to your life from this surgery?
______________ ______________ ______________

6. What is the most common complication after this surgery? ______________________________

7. What is the most important activity after surgery? ______________

8. How soon after surgery do you have to start walking? ______________

9. What is your exercise plan for the first six weeks after surgery? ______________

10. What is your exercise plan for 6 weeks after surgery? ______________

11. What two types of foods will cause the dumping syndrome? ______________ ______________

12. How much protein will you need to take in each day? ______________

13. How much food can you eat at one sitting after surgery? ______________

14. How long does it take for your body to heal the incisions? ______________

15. How much water does you body need each day? ______________

16. How long is your hospital stay? ______________

17. How soon can you start drinking liquids after the surgery? ______________

18. List the four simple sugars: ____________ ____________ ____________ ____________

19. How much simple sugar can you eat without dumping? ________ grams/meal

20. How much fat can you eat without dumping? ________ grams/meal

21. Who is going to be your primary support person? __________________________

22. How many support group meetings will you attend before surgery? __________

Workup Checklist for Surgery

Risk Factors for Heart Disease:

☐ Obesity ☐ Smoking History

☐ Hypertension ☐ Family History

☐ Diabetes ☐ HgbA1C < 8.0

☐ Hyperlipidemia Cholesterol ____ Triglycerides ____

Need for a Cardiology Evaluation? Y/N

Asthma

Ever Hospitalized? Y/N

Ever treated with oral or IV steroids Y/N

Use Inhaler for Rescue? Y/N

How many times a week? ____

Need for a pulmonology consult? Y/N

Need for spirometry Y/N

Workup Checklist for Surgery

Sleep Apnea

- ☐ Snoring
- ☐ Daytime somnolence
- ☐ Early fatigue
- ☐ Morning Headaches
- ☐ Hypertension
- ☐ Apneic episodes

CPAP machine   Setting ____

Need for a sleep study   Y/N

Biliary Disease

- ☐ Pain after fatty meals
- ☐ Pain under right ribcage
- ☐ Dyspeptic symptoms
- ☐ Sonogram with gallstones
- ☐ Family History of gallstones
- ☐ Previous gallbladder operation

Need for gallbladder removal   Y / N

Workup Checklist for Surgery

Risk of blood clots

- ☐ Male
- ☐ BMI > 60
- ☐ Smoking
- ☐ Previous clots
- ☐ Varicose veins
- ☐ Venous stasis disease
- ☐ Surgery > 1 hr
- ☐ Pelvic or knee surgery
- ☐ Limited mobility pre op or post op
- ☐ Birth control pills
- ☐ Hormone replacement therapy

Need for a vena cava filter Y/N

Reflux Disease

- ☐ Indigestion or heartburn after meals
- ☐ Indigestion or heartburn at night
- ☐ Dyspeptic symptoms
- ☐ Sour taste in your mouth
- ☐ Waking with choking or cough
- ☐ Waking with a sore throat

Need for upper endoscopy Y/N

H. Pylori biopsy + / -

Workup Checklist for Surgery

Colonoscopy

- ☐ Age > 50
- ☐ History of polyps
- ☐ Blood in stool
- ☐ Black tarry stools
- ☐ Diarrhea
- ☐ Diverticulitis
- ☐ Family history of colon cancer

Need for a colonoscopy Y / N

Lab work

- ☐ CBC WBC _____ Hgb _____
- ☐ CMP
- ☐ Prealbumin _____
- ☐ HgbA1C _____
- ☐ Cholesterol HDL _____ LDL _____ VLDL _____
- ☐ Triglycerides ________
- ☐ H. Pylori antigen + / -

Preoperative Consultations

☐ Cardiac Stress Evaluation Date: ________
Dr. ______________

☐ Pulmonary Consultation Date: ________
Dr. ______________

☐ Sleep Study Date: ________
CPAP Setting _____
Dr. ______________

☐ Mental Health eval Date: ________
Dr. ______________

☐ Gastroenterology Consultation

☐ EGD Date: ________
H. Pylori +/-

☐ Colonoscopy Date: ________
Dr. ______________

☐ Dietary Consultations Date: ______________

☐ Gallbladder Sonogram Date: ______________

☐ Spirometry Date: ______________

☐ Labwork: Date: ______________

CBC, CMP, Iron, folate, B12, Mg, Phos, Prealbumin
HgbA1C, Thyroid panel, Calcium, Vit D, Lipid panel

Discharge Instructions

Pre-operative medications:

If you were on high blood pressure medications, water pills (diuretics like maxide, hydrochlorothiazide, dyazide, etc.) or diabetic medications, ask whether you should restart these after surgery. Make an appointment to see your primary care physician in two weeks, so they can determine whether you still need these medications after surgery. Otherwise you can take any other medications you were on before surgery.

Post-operative medications:

(prescriptions that may be provided by your doctor)

A hydrocodone liquid is prescribed for pain. You can take one to two teaspoons at six-hour intervals, as needed, for discomfort. This medication can cause nausea, so call early if nausea occurs.

Nausea sometimes occurs for other reasons as well, so a prescription for phenergan, an anti-nausea suppository is given to you. Fill the prescription only if you need it.

Everyone should take ranitidine 150 mg by mouth twice a day for the first six weeks. This is a medicine to decrease acid in the pouch and prevent ulcers and scarring in the pouch.

After your first week at home, start a sugar-free chewable multivitamin like Bugs Bunny® or Flintstone's® twice a day. After six weeks you can take any multivitamin you like, but be sure it is smaller than an M&M in diameter. You will also want to take a B-complex supplement.

After six weeks, start taking two Tums twice a day to increase your calcium intake.

Discharge Instructions

Activity:

The risk of blood clots can last for two to three weeks, so remember to continue walking several times a day. Also, laying down for extended periods of time can lead to fever or pneumonia, so try to spend most of the day sitting up in a chair rather than lying down. If you have a long drive home, stop every one or two hours and walk for five minutes.

You can begin to drive short distances when you are off pain medications no longer have discomfort in your incision. Typically this occurs in about two weeks.

Do not lift anything over ten pounds or you risk developing a hernia in the incision. This would require surgical repair in the future. Your incision gains strength within about six weeks, and then you can become more active.

Exercise:

You must exercise to lose weight. Not exercising means your weight loss will be only marginal. To help prevent blood clots and to help prevent hernias, walking is the recommended exercise. Start with four trips a day. Walk at least fifty (50) yards each trip. This means that walking in the house, to and from the kitchen or bathroom, is not enough. Get outside and walk up and down the block, or go to a store or mall and walk there. Increase the length of each walking trip every day. At the time of your six-week visit, your goal should be to walk one mile each trip, or four miles per day.

Discharge Instructions

Diet:

Follow the dietician's instructions. Remember that it is easy to become dehydrated, so keep a large cup of water with you at all times and sip from it frequently. Sixty-four ounces per day is your minimum fluid intake requirement. Also remember that the goal of surgery is to help you change the way you eat. Only a change in your eating habits leads to weight loss.

Wound Care:

It is not uncommon for your incision to leak a little fluid or even some blood in small amounts. Call if warmth and an increasing area of redness appear around the area of incision. Please shower over the incision daily, allowing water and soap to run over the incision.

You should try to wear the binder for the first two weeks to support the incision, and place gauze pads over the incision to protect it from the binder. The little white tapes will start to peel in a week or two. As the edges peel up, you can pull them off.

Follow-up:

It is critical to follow-up at the scheduled intervals. Your first visit is in two weeks. If you are experiencing any difficulties, call your surgeon first. If you begin to experience problems early in the day, go ahead and call that morning. Problems are always easier to solve when they are addressed early in the day. It is also easier to get things done during daytime hours. Do not feel as if you will inconvenience anyone; our concern is your well-being. If you call after 5:00 pm, the answering service will give you instructions on how to page me, and I will call you back.

Discharge Instructions

It sometimes takes time to get the message from one person to the next, so do not get worried if you are not called back within the first thirty minutes or so. If you feel there is an immediate life-threatening emergency, call 911 or go to the nearest emergency center.

Prescriptions:

Hydrocodone Elixir: One to two teaspoons by mouth on six-hour intervals as needed for pain.

Phenergan: Suppository form taken on six-hour intervals as needed for nausea. Fill this prescription only if you need it, and call your doctor if you are having nausea.

Ranitidine: Take one tablet by mouth twice a day. These help prevent ulcers and allow the pouch to heal.

Remember - any pills bigger than a plain M&M must cut or crushed. For any medications that come as capsules - capsules do not dissolve after your surgery and will pass through unopened. Open medications that come as capsules and add the medication to your food.

Laparoscopic Surgery

The field of surgery is undergoing a revolution and an evolution. Minimally invasive or laparoscopic techniques are being developed for every kind of surgery performed. Patients often have the choice of an open versus a laparoscopic approach, and this includes patients interested in the band, the sleeve, and the Roux en Y gastric bypass.

Minimally invasive techniques involve small incisions with small tubes that are placed across the abdominal wall and into the abdominal space. The abdominal space is filled with an inert gas that stretches the abdominal wall off the organs to create a "dome" to work in. A miniature camera allows the surgeon to see inside, and specialized instruments allow the surgeon to pick up, cut, and sew.

These techniques require not just special equipment and training, but also special abilities. The camera produces a two-dimensional image, so a surgeon has to develop a three-dimensional model in his/her mind that allows him/her to understand what is where in the abdomen. Not every surgeon possesses the ability to do this.

The laparoscopic Roux en Y gastric bypass is considered the most difficult laparoscopic abdominal surgery to perform. How do you know your surgeon is capable of performing this surgery safely? By performing two other operations, a surgeon generally develops laparoscopic skills needed to perform this surgery. The laparoscopic fundoplication surgery teaches the surgeon to operate on the stomach.

Laparoscopic colon resections teach the surgeon to cut and sew on the bowel and to control its blood supply. If your surgeon is trained to do these operations, he/she most likely possesses the ability to learn the laparoscopic Roux en Y. If your surgeon performs the laparoscopic Roux en Y, but not these other operations, you may want to reconsider the laparoscopic approach with that surgeon.

Experience is equally important. Most surgeons are proficient with this procedure after approximately fifty surgeries. If your surgeon has performed fewer than fifteen of these surgeries, he/she may need more experience. If your surgeon has done between fifteen and fifty, then consider how long does it take to finish a laparoscopic Roux en Y? If he/she are able to perform the case in less than three to four hours, then he/she is well on their way to proficiency. Probably the most important factor is the surgeon's experience in performing open Roux en Y procedures. It takes a strong understanding of the open operation, its techniques and complications, to form the basics necessary for the safe laparoscopic approach. A minimum of fifty open cases is recommended.

It is also important to know if the surgeons are performing the same surgery laparoscopically as they perform in their open operations. The procedures should be exactly the same. The risks should be similar, but they do differ between the two approaches. The laparoscopic approach does offer significant improvements over the open technique. There are fewer wound infections and hernias because the incisions are small. There is less pain with the smaller incisions so patients are more comfortable and become more active in a shorter period of time. It also allows patients to return to work sooner and patients generally leave the hospital in one or two days.

Laparoscopic Roux en Y gastric bypass is an excellent operation in the hands of an experienced surgeon, but is difficult to perform. In the hands of an inexperienced surgeon, it may be a more dangerous operation. If your surgeon offers the laparoscopic approach, be sure he/she are appropriately qualified. Your hospital will have strict requirements to determine who is qualified to perform this complex surgery.

Revision Surgery

A certain percentage of patients will fail to either lose enough weight initially or fail to keep the weight off in the long term. Why this happens is a matter of compliance to the dietary changes that surgery is trying to force upon you.

Volume restriction is obtained by creating a small pouch with a small outlet. If you are constantly vomiting, and there are no abnormalities in your pouch or outlet, then you are either overfilling or eating too fast. This puts pressure on the pouch and can either stretch the pouch or, more commonly, stretch the outlet. When you develop greater meal volumes, a major mechanism of weight loss has been destroyed. Because you can now eat more, you are getting more calories in.

The same factors that cause loss of volume restriction cause loss of early satiety. This means that you will feel hungrier and probably eat more often and in increasing amounts. Obviously this will lead to weight gain.

If you continue to eat high calorie/low volume foods, even in the face of dumping for gastric bypass patients, then you are either going to fail to lose weight or regain weight.

I strongly encourage all patients to avoid any carbonated beverages (sodas) due to the damage that occurs to your surgery when you drink them.

Four mechanisms of action are used in weight loss surgery:

1. Volume restriction through formation of a small gastric pouch

2. Early satiety through formation of a narrow outlet from the gastric pouch

3. Malabsorption through bypass of small intestine

4. Avoidance of high calorie/low volume foods through personal effort or as a result of the dumping syndrome.

Depending on the surgery you had, one or more of these effects cause a change in the way you eat. The dietary changes are well described in this book, but if you cannot make the changes, you will not lose weight. If you were poorly educated before your surgery, and did not know how to make these changes, then revision is a possibility after appropriate education. It may not be fair to change the way you have to eat without telling you how to eat, but it happens.

If you have a laparoscopic adjustable gastric band, and you do not get adequate weight loss, you may have had a poor adjustment schedule. If you had a frequent adjustment schedule, but continue to have difficulty losing weight, you can have the band removed. Then, when an appropriate amount of time has passed to allow healing, you can opt for a gastric sleeve operation or a gastric bypass operation. If the band erodes into the stomach for any reason, the surgical technique is most often converted to gastric sleeve or gastric bypass because the recurrent erosion rates for a replacement band are high.

The gastric sleeve operation is the only non-reversible operation currently being performed. It is non-reversible because the extra stomach portion is removed from the body. If you need a revision for better weight loss or for any complication, this will be converted to a gastric bypass, but you will not have as much lower gastric remnant.

If you had a gastric bypass and regained weight or did not lose enough initial weight, some workup may be needed to determine the best revision for you. If the pouch is large or the outlet is dilated, they can both be reduced. Currently, a procedure called Stomaphyx® can be used to re-size the pouch and outlet. It is not a permanent revision, but can serve to re-introduce better volume control and satiety.

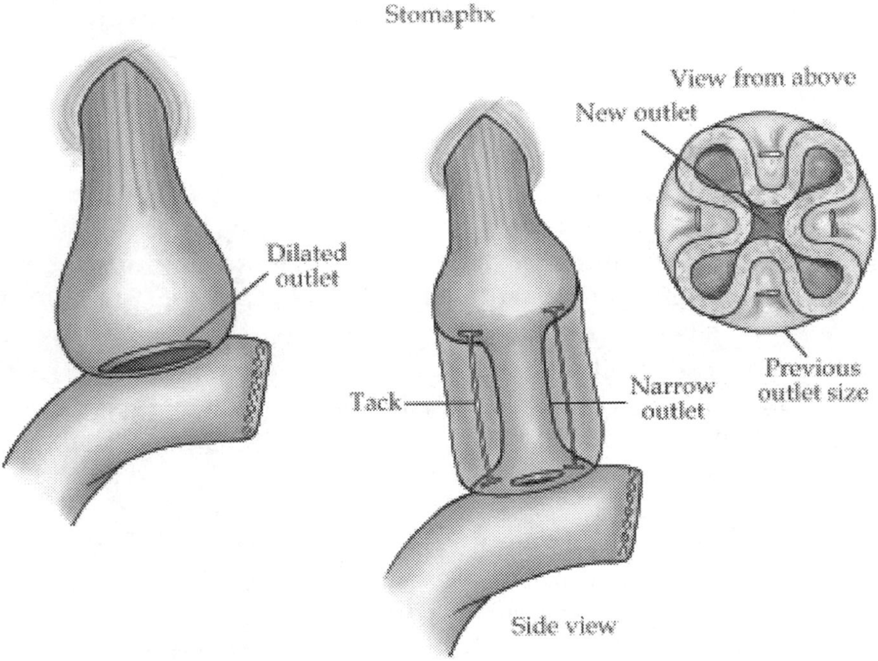

Small plastic tacks are used to pleat the small pouch inward, creating a smaller pouch volume and a narrower outlet.

An advantage of the Stomaphyx® procedure is that it is performed as an endoscopy. No incisions are used to create the changes. The procedure is performed from inside the stomach pouch using a device that fits over an endoscope.

The traditional method to revise a gastric bypass consists of an open or laparoscopic surgery to reduce the pouch size and re-calibrate the outlet to the small bowel. Additional bowel can be bypassed to increase the malabsorption component of the surgery, but there is the increased risk of malnutrition and diarrhea. If you continue to eat the high calorie/low volume foods despite dumping, then either your education was very poor, or you are not very smart. Your education can be improved, but if you continue to eat foods that cause dumping, then the problems are more than surgery alone can fix. A mental health professional may be able to help you improve the anxieties or depression that causes you to eat despite getting sick. Surgery is not a cure-all for every demon that causes you to overeat, but the operation can provide strong incentive to change eating habits that are otherwise too hard to change.

About the Author

Dr. Ihde is a general surgeon in the Dallas/Ft. Worth Metroplex. He obtained a B.S. of Chemistry at Creighton University in 1988. He then attended medical school at the University of Kansas School of Medicine in Kansas City, Kansas. He performed his postgraduate surgical training at the University of Kansas School of Medicine in Wichita, Kansas, under the tutelage of Dr. George Farha. During his surgical training he developed an interest in critical care and nutrition. Additionally, he concentrated on the developing practice of advanced laparoscopic techniques. After participating in a program of open Roux en Y gastric bypass, he developed the laparoscopic program that is now established at three separate hospitals. He is a member of the American Society of Metabolic and Bariatric Surgery. His is a member and has served as an officer of the Texas Association for Bariatric Surgery.

Printed in the United States
By Bookmasters